Health and Poverty

Health and Poverty

Global Health Problems and Solutions

Gijs Walraven

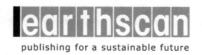

publishing for a sustainable future

London • Washington, DC

To Roz, Ralf and Casper

Earthscan Ltd, Dunstan House, 14a St Cross Street, London EC1N 8XA, UK
Earthscan LLC,1616 P Street, NW, Washington, DC 20036, USA
Earthscan publishes in association with the International Institute for Environment and Development

For more information on Earthscan publications, see www.earthscan.co.uk or write to earthinfo@earthscan.co.uk

ISBN: 978-1-84971-180-7 hardback
ISBN: 978-1-84971-181-4 paperback

Typeset by FiSH Books
Cover design by Clifford Hayes

A catalogue record for this book is available from the British Library

Library of Congress Cataloging-in-Publication Data

Walraven, Gijsbertus Engelinus Laurentius, 1957–
    Health and poverty : global health problems and solutions / Gijs Walraven.
        p. cm.
    Includes bibliographical references and index.
    ISBN 978-1-84971-180-7 (hardback) — ISBN 978-1-84971-181-4 (pbk.) 1. Poverty—Health aspects. 2. Health services accessibility. 3. Equality—Health aspects. 4. World health. I. Title.
    [DNLM: 1. World Health. 2. Healthcare Disparities. 3. Poverty. 4. Primary Health Care. WA 530.1 W221h 2010]
    RA418.5.P6W35 2010
    362.1086'942—dc22

2010019116

At Earthscan we strive to minimize our environmental impacts and carbon footprint through reducing waste, recycling and offsetting our CO_2 emissions, including those created through publication of this book. For more details of our environmental policy, see www.earthscan.co.uk.

Printed and bound in the UK by TJ International, an ISO 14001 accredited company. The paper used is FSC certified.

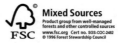

Mixed Sources
Product group from well-managed forests and other controlled sources
www.fsc.org Cert no. SGS-COC-2482
© 1996 Forest Stewardship Council
FSC

Contents

List of Figures, Tables and Boxes

Figures

Tables

Boxes

Foreword

It is a pleasure for me to write this foreword for my colleague and friend Dr Gijs Walraven. His book *Health and Poverty. Global health problems and solutions* gives a new and very human face to the health issues facing poor populations in the developing world today. Dr Walraven's extensive first-hand knowledge of these issues is the concrete basis for his work, and the range of solutions proposed are firmly grounded on tested, practical, and effective interventions. Thanks to this book we come to a better understanding of the complex intrinsic links between health and poverty in poor countries, and of the general field of 'development' as a whole.

This book identifies the health problems that have a disproportionate impact on poor individuals, families and communities in the developing world. The data in Table 1.1 on page 3 dramatically illustrate the differences in life expectancy, maternal and child health and financial investments in health between high and low-income countries. *Health and poverty* also traces the efforts of public health pioneers to remedy the health problems most common among the poor, and breaks new ground by noting that the problems of poverty and illness must be addressed on a regional, cross-border basis and not solely within the geographical boundaries of nation states. Finally, it offers assurances that measures in place and supported by governments and the international community, like health financing, family planning and 'Roll Back Malaria', can contribute to breaking the cycle of poverty and ill-health.

While this book can fit easily in the canon of publications on poverty and illness, it is unique because it is written from a personal perspective by someone who has worked in developing countries for more than 20 years to address sickness among the poor. This thoughtful, practical and personal account moves easily and explains well the relevance of the individual case within the context of the community and the nation. Although a public health professional who is accustomed to diagnosing health problems within the community and putting priority programmes in place to improve health status, Gijs Walraven focuses his work on the afflicted individual, outlining the consequences of illness and death for that individual and his/her family. For those who have come to the study of public health and development after witnessing the problems afflicting the poor, his work will remind each of the origins of his/her commitment and provide assurances that substantial progress has been and can be achieved. Students and practicing development professionals will also find useful the 'Suggestions for Further Reading' sections, which appear at the end of each chapter, and the Glossary, which is placed at the end of this volume.

Grounded in the practical, this book offers concrete solutions to the poverty-disease paradigm. Dr. Walraven argues that the practice of providing inadequate and unequal health care in the developing world is 'unacceptable – economically, ethically, socially and politically,' and affirms that solutions and appropriate financing can be put in place and should be directed to strengthen health systems at all levels.

This work, based on study, experience and conviction, is informative and comprehensive, and deserves to be read and discussed by anyone interested in global health.

Zahra Aga Khan

Acknowledgements

The aim of this book is to stimulate interest in global health issues for a general audience. It uses a format – stories of patients and people, historical context of the problem, why it is still a problem now for poor people and in poor countries, and what can be done about it – that, I hope, grasps and engages the reader. Some of the stories were written 15–20 years ago when I was a young tropical doctor in Sumve, a rural district hospital in Tanzania. Other 'vignettes' are based on experiences while living and working as a clinical epidemiologist in Farafenni, The Gambia, and the most recent ones build on encounters during my visits to communities and health facilities in Central and South Asia. I want to acknowledge all those people with whom I worked during these times – patients, community health leaders, fellow health care providers, researchers and managers – and who inspired me to write this book.

I am very grateful to the patients, their guardians or relatives, who have allowed me to describe the cases in this book. I have changed names and circumstantial details to preserve anonymity as much as possible, but have tried to retain the colour and the character of the people I describe and my encounters with them.

I thank friends and colleagues, old and new, for their great help. Robert Beaglehole, Wil Dolmans, Geert Tom Heikens, Allan Hill, Abid Hussain, Sulaiman Ladhani, Keith McAdam, Asif Merchant, David Molyneux, Najmuddin Najm, Gorik Ooms, Carine Ronsmans and Rengaswamy Sankaranarayanan have given helpful comments on individual chapters. I was privileged to receive advice from Henri van Asten, Jennifer Blum, Nazneen Kanji, David Moore, Angus Nicoll, Jos van Roosmalen, Maarten Schim van der Loeff and John Tomaro who read a draft or drafts of the whole book. I would especially like to thank Rosalind Coleman and Geoffrey Targett, who have given me unstinting support and feedback from the moment they were given a draft of the first chapter that I had written. There will be flaws – and they are mine.

The book brings together information that people all over the world have collected and analysed. The statistics come from a range of sources, in particular the United Nations agencies and the World Bank. I would like to acknowledge Olivier Beerhalter, who used these statistical data to produce the maps that you will find in this book. I would also like to thank Josiane Marti for her excellent administrative help.

Finally, I thank Tim Hardwick at Earthscan for taking on the book's publication, and the Earthscan team for their help during its preparation.

Gijs Walraven,
April 2010

1
The poor have no face, no voice

It is a trite saying that one half of the world knows not how the other lives. Who can say what sores might be healed, what hurts solved, were the doings of each half of the world's inhabitants understood and appreciated by the other?

Mahatma Ghandi, 1906

Health and inequity

There is simply no doubt about it: health and poverty are inextricably linked; and both have an effect on each other. Because of this, increasing health – whether through informational campaigns and prevention, through increased access to medication or through other means – is a sure way to reduce poverty.

'A Dollar a Day. Finding solutions to poverty' website, 2009
(www. library.thinkquest.org/05aug/00282/over_causes.htm.)

Although risk factors for ill health change over time, they tend to be clustered disproportionally at the lower end of the social hierarchy – whether between or within countries. The better-off, more educated, more powerful and richer countries as well as wealthier sections within countries have much greater capacity to maintain and improve their health than do the less well-off. This pattern has been well documented across the ages.

Until the 19th century, deaths of infants, children and mothers were commonplace worldwide. Poor nourishment left most people stunted by today's standards. Communicable diseases such as smallpox, measles and tuberculosis decimated entire communities and left many people scarred and crippled. Life expectancy was low throughout the world. Women in England had the world's highest life expectancy between 1600 and 1840, but even this fluctuated between 35 and 45 years, half of what it is today. The overall picture has changed rapidly and dramatically since the mid-19th century. The medical community brought many communicable diseases under control, and even eradicated smallpox; better nutrition and overall health and living conditions lowered mortality rates for everyone, especially children; and life expectancy increased dramatically. After 1840, the upward trend in global life expectancy proceeded at a surprisingly sustained and uniform rate of increase of 2.5 years per decade for the next 160 years. By 1900, the highest average life expectancy just surpassed 60 years, and now, in 2010, it exceeds 80 years. However, the gains in health and life expectancy have not been uniform around the globe.

Between 1960 and 2007, average overall life expectancy at birth rose from 69 to 79 years in the high-income countries, from 36 to 73 years in China, from 56 to 72 years in Latin America and the Caribbean, and from 44 to 64 years in South Asia. However, in sub-Saharan Africa, average life expectancy only rose from 40 to 46 years, and is therefore more than three decades lower than in the rich countries. What is not well-known is the large variation within regions or (sub-)continents. In sub-Saharan Africa today, children born in Sierra Leone have a life expectancy of 42 years while this stands at 73 years in Mauritius; in South Asia a child born in Afghanistan has a life expectancy of 44 years while it is 72 years in Sri Lanka. Swaziland, Angola and Zambia have life expectancies of just over 40 years, while the life expectancy in countries such as Japan, Australia, Canada, France, Sweden and Switzerland is more than 80 years. A child born in Ethiopia or Afghanistan today has a 20 per cent chance of dying before the age of five compared with a less than 1 per cent chance for a child born in North America or Western Europe. A woman's risk of death in childbirth is around 10 per 100,000 live births in rich countries, but the average is 790 per 100,000 live births in poor countries (see Table 1.1). These inequalities in health indicators can be defined as health inequities: these differences in health are unnecessary, unfair and unjust.

When country-level data are disaggregated to examine the fate of different groups within societies, similarly disturbing health inequities are apparent. Even in rich countries such as Finland, The Netherlands, the UK and the US, the relatively poor die 5–15 years before the rich. Although we tend to assume that the differences between the rich and the poor have been diminishing in rich countries, during the last few decades the health differences between these groups have increased. The gulf between the lives and experience of the rich and the relatively poor, the well educated and the less educated, and different racial and ethnic groups, call into question the humanity, morality and values of modern rich societies.

But the inequities are even sharper within poor countries. Studies from many poor countries show that the poorest 20 per cent ('quintile') of the population fares far worse than the richest 20 per cent on a range of health outcomes, including child mortality and nutritional status. On average a child in the poorest 20 per cent is twice as likely to die before the age of five as a child in the richest 20 per cent, but in some countries the risk is up to five times as high. The disparity is similar for maternal nutrition, with women in the poorest 20 per cent almost twice as likely to be undernourished as those in the richest 20 per cent.

Table 1.1 *Key health and finance related development data and statistics, comparing high-income and low-income countries*

Indicator	High-income countries	Low-income countries
Population	1.068 billion	0.972 billion
Life expectancy at birth	79 years	59 years
Fertility rate (births per woman)	1.8	4.0
Maternal mortality ratio (per 100,000 live births)	10	790
Births attended by skilled health staff (% of total)	99	43
Under-5 mortality rate (per 1000)	7	120
Immunization, measles (% of children aged 12–23 months)	93	78
Prevalence of HIV, total (% of population aged 15–49)	0.3	2.3
Aggregate GDP	US$43,189 billion	US$558 billion
GDP per person	US$40,439	US$584
Public health expenditure per person	6–8% of GDP/US$2426–3,235	1–2% of GDP/US$6–12

Source: World Development Indicators database, April 2009. GDP = gross domestic product

So, the poor suffer worse health and die younger. But for poor people especially, health is also an extremely important economic asset. Their livelihoods depend on it. When a poor person becomes ill or injured, the entire household can become trapped in a downward spiral of lost income and high health care costs. The cascading effects may also include diverting time from generating an income or from schooling to care for the sick. And illness in the family may force the sale of assets – livestock or land required for livelihoods. More prone to disease and with limited access to health care and social insurance, poor people are more vulnerable to this downward spiral. Good health contributes to development. Healthier workers are more productive, earn higher wages and miss fewer days of work than those who are ill. Increased labour productivity in turn creates incentives for investment.

Healthy children have better cognitive potential. As health improves, rates of absenteeism and early school drop-outs fall, and children learn better, leading to a growth in human capital. Improvements in both health and education can contribute to lower rates of fertility and mortality. After a delay, fertility usually falls faster than mortality, slowing population growth and reducing the 'dependency factor' (the ratio of dependents to active workers). This 'demographic dividend' has been shown to be an important source of per capita growth for poor countries; it is also of great importance at the household level of poor families. The poor tend to have more children, and invest less in the education and health of each child. With better health and education, family size declines. Children are more inclined to escape the cognitive and physical consequences of childhood illnesses and to do better at school. They are less likely to suffer disability and impairment in later life, and are less likely to face catastrophic health expenditures and more likely to achieve their earning potential. Then, as healthy adults, they have more resources to invest in the care, health and education of their own children. Health improvements have intergenerational spill-over effects; health is a foundation for prosperity both at the micro- and macro-economic level.

Why are there health gaps between the rich and the poor?

To me this seems a shocking and monstrous inequity of very considerable proportions that, simply because of relative affluence, I should be living when others have died, that I should remain healthy when illness and death beset millions of others.

Edwin Cameron, 2000

Poverty makes people more vulnerable to disease. The World Bank estimated that in 2005 1.4 billion people lived on less than $1.25 a day, the new official cut-off point for extreme poverty, while another 1.2 billion lived on between $1.25 and $2 a day. Roughly 1 billion people still lived on less than 1 dollar a day, the so-called 'bottom billion'. Some 40 per cent of people in South Asia (or around 600 million people) and half of the people in sub-Saharan Africa (around 380 million people) live on $1.25 a day or less. The majority of them typically lack access to safe drinking water and adequate sanitation, food, education, employment, health information and professional health care. Almost half the people in sub-Saharan Africa cannot obtain essential drugs, and similarly less than half of women giving birth are assisted by skilled birth attendants. A review of 42 poor countries, which account for 90 per cent of global child deaths, showed that only 2 out of 9 key interventions reached more than half of all children. For example, many of these countries experienced little increase in immunization coverage between 1990 and 2005, and in 2005 only 75 per cent of children aged 12–23 months were vaccinated against the common childhood infections, compared to 95 per cent for rich countries. Several factors other than low-income prevent people in poor countries from accessing appropriate care, namely services, clients and institutions. *Service factors* include the high costs of care and transportation, distances to services and the time needed to reach them, poor quality care, inappropriate care, negative staff attitudes and cultural and linguistic differences. *Client factors* include social and cultural constraints, especially for women who have limited mobility and lower incomes and wealth, and greater time burdens because of their assigned roles within the family, as well as local (mis)perceptions of illness. The poor in general have often limited information about their health needs and rights and about the availability of services.

Institutional factors include issues such as not enough attention paid to health promotion and disease prevention, local treatment norms, stigma and discrimination by health providers, and a lack of voice for the poor when it comes to decision making, including health budgets.

Health and the millennium development goals

> *The millennium development goals can be met by 2015, but only if all involved break with business as usual and dramatically accelerate and scale up action now.*
>
> Kofi Annan, 2005

Health is now higher on the international agenda than ever before; concern for the health of poor people has become a central issue in development. The nations of the world have agreed that enjoying the highest attainable standard of health is one of the fundamental rights of every human being without distinction of race, religion, political belief and economic or social condition. At the Millennium Summit in September 2000 the largest gathering of world leaders in history adopted the United Nations Millennium Declaration, committing their nations to a new global partnership to reduce poverty and to set out a number of time-bound targets, all with a deadline of 2015. These commitments underpin the eight Millennium Development Goals; three are directly health related and call for a two-thirds reduction in child mortality, a three-quarters reduction in maternal mortality, and a halt to the spread of HIV/AIDS, malaria and other diseases. Box 1.1 lists the 8 goals and 18 targets that are bold commitments to achieve sustainable development for the world's poorest people.

The first seven Millennium Development Goals call for sharp reductions in poverty, disease and environmental degradation. The eighth goal is essentially a commitment to a global partnership, a pact between rich and poor countries to work together to achieve the first seven goals. This also includes a call to ensure that poor countries have access to affordable essential drugs. The Millennium Development Goals recognize that extreme poverty has many dimensions, not only low income, but also vulnerability to disease, exclusion from education, the gnawing presence of hunger and undernutrition, lack of access to basic amenities such as safe water, adequate sanitation and shelter, and environmental degradation such as deforestation and land erosion that threatens lives and livelihoods. While only three goals relate directly to health, health is central to achieving all eight goals, especially those related to reducing/eliminating extreme poverty and hunger, and promoting gender equality. However, despite the priority concern for health at the international level and the unprecedented attention and resources, progress to achieve the health related Millennium Development Goals has so far been too slow for most targets to be met by 2015. In addition, even where there is progress, it is possible for countries to neglect equity in the race to achieve the set goals and

Box 1.1 *The Millennium Development Goals and Targets*

1	Eradicate extreme poverty and hunger	• Halve, between 1990 and 2015, the proportion of people whose income is less than one dollar a day • Halve, between 1990 and 2015, the proportion of people who suffer from hunger
2	Achieve universal primary education	• Ensure that by 2015 children everywhere, boys and girls alike, will be able to complete a full course of primary education
3	Promote gender equality and empower women	• Eliminate gender disparity in primary and secondary education, preferably by 2005, and to all levels of education no later than 2015
4	Reduce child mortality	• Reduce by two-thirds, between 1990 and 2015, the under-five mortality rate
5	Improve maternal health	• Reduce by three-quarters, between 1990 and 2015, the maternal mortality ratio
6	Combat HIV/AIDS, malaria and other diseases	• Have halted by 2015 and begun to reverse the spread of HIV/AIDS • Have halted by 2015 and begun to reverse the incidence of malaria and other major diseases
7	Ensure environmental sustainability	• Integrate the principles of sustainable development into country policies and programmes and reverse the loss of environmental resources • Half by 2015 the proportion of people without sustainable access to safe drinking water and basic sanitation • By 2020 to have achieved a significant improvement in lives of at least 100 million slum dwellers
8	Develop a global partnership for development	• Address the special needs of the least developed countries, landlocked countries and small island developing states • Develop further an open, rule-based, predictable, non-discriminatory trading and financial system • Deal comprehensively with developing countries' debts • In cooperation with pharmaceutical companies, provide access to affordable essential drugs in developing countries • In cooperation with the private sector, make available benefits of new technologies, especially information and communication

targets. Given that the poorest populations tend also to be the hardest to reach, and hold marginal political weight, there is often little incentive for governments to prioritize their needs. The measurement of targets across the wealth quintiles in addition to national averages is in this respect very important. An increasingly common measure of equity is the ratio of indicators in the poorest 20 per cent of the population to the richest 20 per cent, the so-called quintile ratio.

Global health

'Global health' has recently become a fashionable term, but what does global health mean? It can be seen as any health problem that goes beyond national borders, and embraces old and emerging diseases. The World Health Organization states on its website that: 'health is a shared responsibility, involving equitable access to essential care and collective defence against transnational threats.' There are two elements in this description: a globally shared responsibility for the health of all people, and global disease threats posed by 'things' that can cross borders. Although the 'things' are more than infectious diseases, it is the infectious diseases that provide the most visible and explicit examples of why shared vulnerability and taking responsibility for the health of all people is important. Uncontrolled epidemics that might become pandemics by moving from poor countries to rich countries motivate the more wealthy to help poor people because the more wealthy do not want to get poor people's diseases. It is probably not a coincidence that development assistance for health seems to focus on infectious diseases disproportionately. However, the right to the highest attainable standard of health for all is increasingly becoming the implicitly agreed objective of the new social movement that is global health and goes well beyond a willingness to tackle global threats posed by infectious diseases. It wants to ensure that there is equal attention and solidarity for non-infectious diseases.

Global health should therefore also address maternal mortality, undernutrition, obesity, tobacco control, injury prevention and the health consequences of stress, urbanization, occupational hazards and global warming. As Jeffrey Koplan and others have recently emphasized 'the global in global health refers to the scope of the problems, not their location'. Global health has to embrace the full breadth of important health threats, and therefore incorporate as well, for example, paying attention to the training and distribution of the global health care workforce. It is also about shared, mutual responsibility and real partnerships, a pooling of experience and knowledge, and a two-way flow between rich and poor countries. And it is about being multi-disciplinary, with contributions from biomedicine, epidemiology, public health, demography, anthropology, history, economics, political science, law, engineering, geography, informatics and philosophy. Koplan and others proposed the following definition: 'global health is an area for study, research, and practice that places a priority on improving health and achieving equity in health for all people worldwide. Global health emphasizes transnational health issues, determinants and solutions; involves many disciplines within and beyond the health sciences and promotes interdisciplinary collaboration; and is a synthesis of population-based prevention with individual-level clinical care.'

William Easterly, an economics professor at New York University, is probably one of the most outspoken sceptics of foreign aid. In *The White Man's Burden* (the title referring to the famous poem by Rudyard Kipling), Easterly distinguishes two types of foreign aid donors: 'Planners', who believe in imposing top-down big plans on poor countries (including the Millennium Development Goals), and 'Searchers', who look for bottom-up solutions to specific needs. Planners are portrayed as utopian and arrogant – best summed up as: 'We – in the West – know best what is good for the Rest' – while Searchers, according to Easterly, have a much better chance of succeeding as they are more focused on realistic interventions with sufficient understanding and respect for the efforts of people themselves and their communities. In the chapter 'The Healers: Triumph and Tragedy' Easterly argues that health is the area where foreign aid has enjoyed its most noticeable successes. He explains that this is because health is an area where the needs and wants of the poor are obvious, the outcomes are visible, well-defined and measurable (increasing the chances that the Searchers are in charge) and coincide with the poor's needs while having political support in rich countries.

Over the past decade, global health initiatives have become a prominent part of the international aid architecture, bringing new resources, political commitment, and more attention to international health issues. Funding for development assistance for health has quadrupled from $5.6 billion in 1990 to $21.8 billion in 2007. At the same time, the availability of the sophisticated arsenal of tools and technologies for preventing and curing disease tends to vary inversely with the need for it; the best care tends to go to those who need it least. The global health community that strives to achieve the highest attainable standard of health for all is fragmented. It allows damaging competition between AIDS and/or malaria and/or tuberculosis (the main targets in Millennium Development Goal 6) versus all other diseases, child survival (Millennium Development Goal 4) versus maternal health (Millennium Development Goal 5), the Millennium Development Goals versus the Non-Millennium Development Goals (such as reproductive health, chronic non-communicable diseases, mental health and injuries), and vertical global health initiatives (such as the Global Fund to fight AIDS, Tuberculosis and Malaria and the Global Alliance for Vaccines and Immunizations) versus health systems and comprehensive primary health care.

This book

This book tells the stories of those with health-related problems, provides for an historical context of the particular problem, argues why it is still a problem now for poor people and in poor countries, and describes what can be done about it. The aim of the book is to give examples of diseases and problems related to health that disproportionally impact the poor, and to give their experiences 'a human face'. It includes problems related to infectious diseases such as malaria (Chapter 2), tuberculosis and HIV (Chapter 3), the neglected tropical diseases (Chapter 8), but also non-communicable diseases such as hypertension and diabetes (Chapter 10), as well as 'communicable non-communicable disease' (cervical cancer in Chapter 6). Differences in health status are also the result of differential exposure to health risks, also called the social determinants of health. Many of these differences are associated with poverty and discussed in a number of chapters in this book, including those on safe motherhood (Chapter 4), family planning (Chapter 5), water and sanitation (Chapter 7), and undernutrition (Chapter 9). This book also includes chapters that look at barriers to access to health care, such as the chapters on health financing (Chapter 11), cross-border health care (Chapter 12) and comprehensive primary health care and health systems (Chapter 13).

I hope this book generates a feeling of optimism about the real possibility that exists now to achieve the highest attainable standard of health for all. As one can read in this book, there are appropriate and ready interventions including new technologies available that prevent and treat diseases that affect the poor disproportionally. Consensus is gathering on the importance of the social determinants of health and how these can be addressed, on strengthening primary health care systems and making these comprehensive, on the importance of the continuum of care, and on integrated health prevention and treatment packages in communities. The title of this introductory chapter refers to the poor having no face and little voice, and this contributes to inequity in health and health care. The stories of Lamin, Pendo, Kaddy, Maimuna, Ramesh, Neelum, Sifat, Ousman, Hassan, Mariama, Helena and Sanam provide for some of these faces and voices. This book also tries to convey the message that striving towards equity in health and health care is a must as inadequate and unequal health care is unacceptable: economically, ethically, socially and politically. It is up to us to respond to the faces and voices in this book.

With the wealth and knowledge that the world has today, and if we can solve the problem of fragmentation that divides the global health community, we can get much closer to achieving the health related Millennium Development Goals by 2015 as well as making progress towards achieving the 'Non-Millennium Development Goals' such as reproductive health and the chronic non-communicable diseases, and the wider 'best attainable health for all' goal than was thought possible only a few years ago. This book gives examples of what can be done, and I hope also conveys the message that we cannot say anymore that we do not know how to do it, nor that we cannot afford to do it, nor that we do not have reason to do it.

Sources and suggestions for further reading

The second edition of *Disease Control Priorities in Developing Countries* (a co-publication of Oxford University Press and the World Bank, 2006) by Dean Jamison and others was a major source of information and inspiration both for this chapter and the book as a whole, as well as the 'back-up' material in *Global Burden of Disease and Risk Factors* by Alan D. Lopez and colleagues, and the short summary document *Priorities in Health* also by Dean Jamison (both these books were also published by Oxford University Press/World Bank in 2006). Timothy Evans et al.'s *Challenging Inequities in Health* opens the door to a debate on the problem as well as how to reduce health inequities (Oxford University Press, New York, 2001). I also consulted *Poverty and Health* published by the Organisation for Economic Co-operation and Development (OECD) and the World Health Organization (Paris, 2003). In a 2006 TED (short for Technology, Entertainment and Design) talk Hans Rosling presented, in a highly entertaining and at the same time original manner, the variation of child survival over time between and within countries against average income per capita (see www.ted.com/talks/hans_rosling_shows_the_best_stats_you_ve_ever_seen.html).

For readers interested in understanding the problem of inequality/inequity in affluent societies Richard Wilkinson's book *The Impact of Inequality: How to make Sick Societies Healthier* (The New Press, New York, 2005) is highly recommended. Richard Wilkinson and Kate Pickett make the case in *The Spirit Level – Why Equality is Better for Everyone* that it is not only the poor in any given country who suffer from inequality, but also the bulk of that country's population (Allen Lane, 2009; Penguin, 2010). The United Nations Millennium Development Goals website (www.un.org/millenniumgoals/) provides much information about the goals and targets, progress to date, as well as gaps and issues. For the thinking on the development of a global health definition please see Jeffrey Koplan and others' viewpoint paper 'Towards a common definition of global health' (*The Lancet* 2009; 373: 1993–5) and Richard Horton's article on 'Global science and social movements: Towards a rational politics of global health' in *International Health* (2009; 1: 26–30). William Easterly's *The White Man's Burden. Why the West's efforts to Aid the Rest Have Done so Much Ill and so Little Good* (Penguin, New York, 2006) is – even if one does not agree with all his ideas and observations – essential reading material for those involved in development cooperation as it is an eye-opener with a lot of food for thought. Dambisa Moyo's *Dead Aid: Why Aid is Not Working and How There is a Better Way for Africa* (Farrar, Straus and Giroux, New York, 2009) is another book in the same category and offers proposals for poor countries to finance development, instead of relying on foreign aid.

2
Roll back malaria

Malaria, long sleeping in the blood
leaps in an adder's fashion, suddenly –
the body unprepared and unattended …

Dorothy Livesay, 1983

Lamin

It is October 1997 in Farafenni, rural Gambia, West-Africa, and the rains are good – good for the crops – and the farmers are hoping for a bumper rice and groundnut harvest. But rain also brings malaria. Lamin, the two-year-old son of Fatou, a nurse assistant at the hospital, was admitted last night to the paediatric ward. He had been treated two weeks ago for malaria but Lamin had a high fever again yesterday afternoon, which Fatou treated with chloroquine, as well as paracetamol and tepid sponging to bring the fever down. Later Lamin vomited and had two episodes of diarrhoea, and when he started having convulsions Fatou immediately brought him to the hospital. Upon arrival, Lamin is unrousable and floppy, and has a high fever. He is clinically anaemic, and I find he has an enlarged spleen upon palpation. The blood film shows a high number of malaria parasites in the red blood cells, and both his haemoglobin and blood sugar are very low. We give Lamin quinine and glucose intravenously, a blood transfusion, a nasogastric tube which helps us to safely feed him, and medicines to prevent further convulsions. Despite these drugs, Lamin has a further two episodes of convulsions. Over the next few days the fever goes down, and a new blood film shows that the malaria parasites have disappeared from his red blood cells, and that his haemoglobin and blood glucose levels have become normal. However, Lamin remains unrousable and reacts abnormally to stimuli in neurological tests. Fatou repeatedly asks me whether Lamin will get better, despite knowing the answer herself very well – possibly, but also possibly not. Two weeks after the day he was admitted Lamin is discharged, but no longer the good-humoured active little boy with sparkly eyes. Lamin dies three months later, and I don't ask Fatou any questions – here a severely handicapped child does not have much of a future.

Roman fever

Malaria has been with us for thousands of years. Hippocrates described cases which included periodic fevers and initial rigors followed by sweating, sometimes associated with an enlarged spleen. Malaria is also to be found in the medical literature of ancient India, where it is referred to as the most dreaded affliction, the 'King of Diseases'. The malady was attributed to the anger of the god Shiva with fevers that were described to return every third ('tertian') or fourth ('quartan') day. Both in this literature and that of the Chinese, tertian and quartan fevers are differentiated and associated with enlarged spleens. The names given to fevers often reflected their supposed origin. 'Malaria' derived from the notion that 'bad' air caused febrile disease, while 'paludism', with its Latin root ('palid' = swamp), acknowledged the historic name given to malaria in Italy – 'swamp fever', 'marsh fever', 'Roman fever'. From about 200 BC until the early 1930s, the area around Rome was a highly endemic malaria area. There was such a close association between malaria and Rome that, in a sense, the Romans viewed the disease in a proprietary fashion – it was their 'Roman fever'. Horace Walpole (Desowitz, p151) in 1740 brought Rome and malaria together in what may be the first reference in the English language to malaria, 'A horrid thing called mal'aria, that comes to Rome every summer and kills one'.

However it was not in Rome, but in Bone, Algeria on 20 October 1880 that the French Army Surgeon Alphonse Laveran (Desowitz, p167) took some blood from a feverish patient, placed a drop on a microscope slide, and saw 'among the red corpuscles, elements that seemed to me to be parasites'. Laveran saw strange crescent-shaped bodies (the gametocytes of the malaria parasite *Plasmodium falciparum*) and, even more astoundingly in a blood slide of another patient on 6 November 1880, some rounded bodies from whose surface 'filaments lashed and sinuously danced' (a living parasite; the flagellated body of the male gametocyte). Laveran was indeed the first to witness the parasite that caused malaria.

It had been Sir Patrick Manson (Desowitz, p35), a Briton who is regarded as the 'father' of tropical medicine, who was the first to demonstrate in 1876 that insects were likely vectors of disease from one human to another. Manson first read about Laveran's results in 1884, but it would be only in 1892 that 'Laveran's' parasites were shown to him. He undertook investigations of his own using sick Indian patients in London. He was struck by the fact that 'the flagellated body never appears or comes into view on the microscope field immediately after the withdrawal of the blood from the patient, but only after the blood has been on the slide for some minutes'. Linked to the fact that malaria was not transmitted directly from one individual to another under normal circumstances, this observation led him to argue that the 'mosquito ... or a similar suctorial insect or insects' were responsible for assisting 'the malarial organism to escape from the human body'. This postulation was published in a paper in 1894, the year in which Manson also met Ronald Ross, a British army surgeon serving in the Indian Medical Services. Inspired by Manson's suggestion that malaria was transmitted through mosquitoes, Ronald Ross returned to Secundarabad, India, determined to prove the hypothesis.

On 20 August 1897, after examining more than a thousand other mosquitoes, Ross saw ' tiny cells with little black spots' among the fibres of the stomach wall of a mosquito that had fed four days earlier on a malarious patient. Ross had found in the stomach wall of an *Anopheles* mosquito the oocysts which are the intermediate stage of the *Plasmodium* life cycle. Ross used bird malaria to show that the development of the parasite in the mosquito was necessary for the transmission of infection by mosquitoes. Working at the same time, Italian investigators Grassi, Bignami and Bastianelli confirmed the need for a similar cycle of development for the human malarias *P. falciparum*, *P. vivax* and *P. malariae*. The discovery that malaria was transmitted by mosquitoes was the beginning of a new era – that of attempts to control malaria. Ross thought that malaria could be controlled by attacking the mosquito where it bred, in fresh water. Ross left India as an authority, having won the Nobel Prize for Medicine in 1902 and having been knighted. He subsequently travelled to many countries preaching the necessity of mosquito control by engineering works that would remove the water, or by oiling the water's surface.

During the first third of the 20th century, the wealthier Western countries, motivated by economic interest, carried out massive antimalarial engineering works. America needed the Panama canal, so General William Crawford Gorgas led the drainage of the swamps and seepages to rid the Canal Zone of malaria and yellow-fever carrying mosquitoes. Perhaps the most monumental of the antimalarial engineering projects was carried out in Mussolini's Italy. During the 1930s, Mussolini, listening to the advice of Italian malariologists, undertook a bold and costly project to make the Pontina, the area west of Rome, safe for human life. An extensive complex of drainage canals was constructed. The Pontina began to dry and the anopheline mosquitoes lost their breeding sites. Malaria transmission was reduced to a point where human settlement became possible.

Although the impressive, large-scale works of Mussolini in the Pontina and of Gorgas in Panama were without any doubt beneficial, they did not help the large numbers of people at risk from malaria in Africa, Asia, tropical America and the Pacific. Large environmental engineering projects are prohibitively expensive for poor counties. And probably more important, it had been Ross himself, working in Sierra Leone in 1899, who had noted that anopheline mosquitoes laid their eggs mainly in puddles, specifically in those that are big enough not to dry up too quickly but small enough not to shelter mosquito- or larvae-eating fish. And Freetown, Sierra Leone's capital, had and has – as have many tropical settlements, especially in sub-Saharan Africa, including Farafenni – lots of puddles and pits when it rains, which cannot be 'dried out' by canals or other engineering works. Ross's method of oiling the puddles was also unsuccessful, and mosquito larvae reappeared whenever the water treatment was stopped.

DDT

This is the DDT era of malariology. For the first time it is economically feasible for nations, however underdeveloped and whatever the climate, to banish malaria completely from their borders

Paul F. Russell, 1955

For poor countries an inexpensive, relatively simple, relatively long-lasting antimalarial measure was needed. That need was thought to have been met with the discovery of dichloro-diphenyl-trichloroethylene (DDT). DDT was first synthesized in 1874. However, it was only in 1939 that its insecticidal properties were discovered. Residual spraying with DDT, which means spraying that leads to DDT 'residing' on the walls where mosquitoes normally land to have a rest, especially after having fed on humans, prevented anopheline mosquitoes from living long enough to become dangerous, and the DDT remained effective for several months after application. The Pontina had been drained in the 1930s and malaria controlled, but not completely eradicated. Malaria was soon to disappear throughout the entire Pontine Marshes after DDT spraying was started. The results of pilot projects with DDT spraying in several countries, albeit mainly in subtropical areas or islands with relatively low malaria transmission, were so good that from 1950 onwards senior malariologists, supported by mathematical models that showed that regular 3–6 monthly spraying with DDT would reduce the mosquito population to too small a size for further transmission of malaria, were advising the widespread use of DDT with the aim of the global eradication of malaria. In 1955, the World Health Organization Assembly endorsed the policy of global eradication.

By the end of the 1960s it became clear that despite an enormous amount of money and effort, mainly from countries where malaria was endemic, that the single-minded effort of DDT spraying to eradicate malaria had failed. Anopheline vectors were becoming resistant to the action of DDT, and changed their behaviour. Lack of political will, inadequate and unsustained funding, bureaucratic procedures, weak health systems, and inadequate and poorly trained staff were additional important factors that contributed to the failure. When DDT stopped killing mosquitoes and other 'pest' insects, public support for the spraying campaigns diminished, and the remaining political and financial commitments waned. In 1972, the global eradication programme was formally declared dead.

At the same time concerns were raised about the ecological consequences of the widespread use of DDT, including persistence in the environment and bioaccumulation and toxic effects. The concerns were that DDT's stable metabolites accumulate in food chains and harm wildlife, including fish. Its use was banned by many countries; but the harmful effects of DDT as used in mosquito control, in comparison with the massive amounts used for agricultural purposes, were often exaggerated. There are suspected human health risks that include the disruption of reproductive and endocrine functions. However, the impact on human health is not proven, certainly not at the levels of DDT detectable as a consequence of indoor spraying, and its regulated use has been increasing again in recent years, bringing some dramatic improvements in malaria control. The World Health Organization's position recognizes a continued role for DDT as the alternative insecticides are costly and less effective (Stockholm Convention on Persistent Organic Pollutants, 1998).There is only limited environmental contamination when DDT is used indoors, but there is a goal to reduce and ultimately eliminate its use by prioritizing research on safe and cost-effective alternative insecticides.

My name is Today

We are guilty of many errors and faults,
but our worst crime is abandoning the children,
neglecting the fountain of life.

Many of the things we need can wait.
The child cannot.

Right now is the time his bones are being formed,
his blood is being made and his senses are being developed.
To him we cannot answer, 'Tomorrow'.
His name is 'Today'.

Gabriela Mistral, 1924

Lamin died of malaria in the centenary year of the discovery of the mosquito transmission of malaria by Ross, and unfortunately the golden jubilee of attempts at malaria eradication has now also passed. Recent estimates suggest that malaria still directly causes about 1 million deaths per year or 3000 deaths a day, and that most of these deaths occur among African children. It is likely that the true number is substantially higher due to indirect effects of the disease on nutrition and other infections. Another estimate puts the number of malaria cases per year at almost 500 million. If anything, malaria has increased over the last 35 years. In malaria-endemic areas, malaria infection in pregnancy is believed to account for up to a quarter of all cases of severe anaemia in mothers and with that it contributes to a substantial number of maternal deaths, as well as neonatal and infant deaths resulting from low birthweight babies. The effect of malaria extends far beyond these direct measures of mortality and disease. Malaria can reduce attendance at school and productivity at work and evidence suggests that the disease can impair intellectual development. The failure of children to fulfil their potential and achieve satisfactory educational levels plays an important part in the intergenerational transmission of poverty. In populations and countries with a large proportion of such children, societal and national development is likely to be affected.

Malaria is the most important parasitic infection in people, and the burden of this large toll is borne by the world's poorest countries. How does the malaria parasite cause fever and why, with similar parasite densities in the blood, do some people recover while others die? Figure 2.1 summarizes the malaria life cycle. Laveran saw gametocytes (the sexual form of the parasite that is ingested by the mosquito when biting humans) 'among the red corpuscles', and Ross saw oocysts in the stomach wall of an *Anopheles* mosquito. Infection of the human host with a *Plasmodium* parasite begins with the bite of an infected *Anopheles* mosquito that inoculates the individual with sporozoites. These motile forms of the parasite rapidly access the blood stream and then the liver, where they invade liver cells. The asymptomatic liver stage of infection lasts one to two weeks, with each sporozoite yielding thousands of merozoites. In the blood stage, the merozoites invade the red blood cells, where

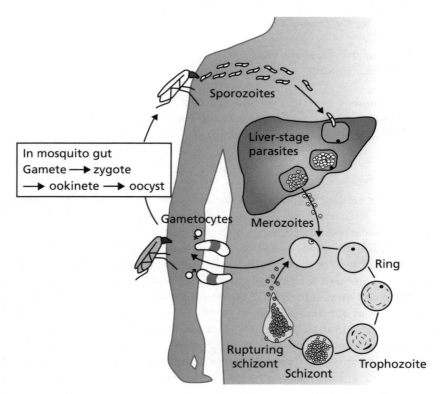

Figure 2.1 *Life cycle of the malaria parasite*

Source: Greenwood. B. et al., *The Lancet* 2005; 365:1487–1498

they grow and multiply. These new merozoites then go on to invade new red blood cells when they burst out of the old cell. The fever is associated with the rupturing of billions of schizonts at about the same time. 'Malaria toxins' are released at this time which trigger a series of reactions in the immune system which, in some people characterized by certain genetic traits, may contribute to subsequent severity, complications and death. The body reacts to the toxins by releasing 'pyrogens' which help destroy the parasites and at the same time trigger the physiological responses that cause fever, including shivering, cold body surface and high pulse. One of these pyrogens, tumour necrosis factor (TNF), is believed to be particularly important in this immune response. However, TNF also seems to contribute to other responses that can make malaria severe.

Lamin suffered from the most fatal form of malaria, cerebral malaria, a syndrome of unrousable coma that occurs in only one of the five Plasmodium parasite species (see Glossary) that cause human malaria. This species, *Plasmodium falciparum*, which causes the majority of infections in Africa, is increasing in several Asian countries, and is responsible for the most severe disease and mortality. Cerebral malaria is characterized by parasite sequestration in small cerebral blood vessels. TNF is thought to promote cerebral malaria by increasing the adhesiveness of the parasitized cells to the lining of the cerebral blood vessels. Nitric oxide is also induced by TNF which, in large amounts, interferes with neurotransmission. TNF may additionally contribute to the pathogenesis of hypoglycaemia (low blood sugar) and severe anaemia, and Lamin had both of these complications as well. Genetic differences in the regulation of TNF by the human host can determine the severity of *falciparum* malaria.

Lamin did not sleep under an insecticide impregnated bed net, the next mosquito control measure that has been propagated on a large scale after the DDT spraying. It was the Farafenni area where it was shown in a community-based controlled research trial in 1992 that sleeping under an insecticide impregnated bed net substantially reduces malaria related child mortality. This success was followed by a national insecticide treated bed net programme in The Gambia, where the impact on child mortality was confirmed in the mid-1990s. Unfortunately, the necessary regular (6-monthly) re-treatment of nets with insecticide proved difficult to sustain, especially if users were required to pay for it. Furthermore, the introduction of insecticide treated materials requires behavioural and socio-economic changes; sleeping under a bed net in a hot environment without electricity and a fan or air conditioning does not happen automatically.

Lamin had been treated in the first and second instances with chloroquine, a drug discovered in the 1940s and used intensively and largely successfully for the treatment and prevention of malaria at the tail-end of the eradication campaign. In 1998 – so in the year after Lamin's death – a paper was published by Jean-François Trape and others, working in neighbouring Senegal, which showed that after the emergence of chloroquine resistance, malaria mortality among children had multiplied up to 6 times over a 12-year period, from 1984 to 1995. In 1999 a group of malaria experts wrote under the title 'Averting a malaria disaster' in the leading medical journal *The Lancet*:

> Malaria morbidity and mortality have been held in check by the widespread availability of cheap and effective antimalarial drugs. The loss of these drugs to resistance may present the single most important threat to the health of people in tropical countries. Chloroquine has been the mainstay of antimalaria drug treatment for the past 40 years, but resistance is now widespread and few countries are unaffected.

A reaction came in the establishment of 'Roll Back Malaria' – an international alliance of more than 90 organizations including the World Health Organization, UNICEF and the World Bank – and intended as the main instrument to reduce malaria mortality. In 2005, in an editorial, *The Lancet* wrote about 'Roll Back Malaria':

> But in the 7 years since its inception, malaria rates have increased and the organization has accumulated an expansive list of missed opportunities and dismal failures.

What has happened since then?

Artemisinin-based combination treatments and long-lasting insecticidal nets

> *Drugs are more often discovered by chance than built by design. At least until very recently, we have known too little about the minute workings of the body, to construct drugs from first principles. But we do now have a grasp of many mechanisms of drug action, understanding why they work even if we found them through good luck.*
>
> Adam Zeman, 2008

Combination therapy with drugs with different modes of action is now the preferred approach to malaria treatment to inhibit the emergence and spread of parasites resistant to one component of the drug therapy. The most widely promoted combinations are artemisinin-based combination treatments. *Artemisia annua*, the shrub from which artemisinin can be isolated, has been used by Chinese herbalists for more than two thousand years in the treatment of many illnesses. Its antimalarial application was first described in the 4th century. In 1967 Mao Tse-Tung's government ordered the systematic examination of the traditional Chinese pharmacopeia that led to the isolation of the compound *qinghaosu*, or artemisinin in 1972. This story is not dissimilar to the one of quinine, the drug that was used to treat Lamin's cerebral malaria and isolated around 1800 in South America from the *Cinchona* bark or 'fever bark tree'. The cinchona bark had also been used to treat fevers for several centuries before the isolation of the active ingredient. Unfortunately the discovery of *qinghaosu* remained unknown to the rest of the world for many years after its discovery. There are now, however, good efficacy and effectiveness data supporting several artemisinin-based combination treatments.

Many deaths from malaria occur in the community before any contact is made with the formal health sector. Several developments have the potential to improve this situation. These advances include home-management that provides effective treatment as close to home as possible, the training of shopkeepers who sell drugs, the packaging of drugs and the development of artemisinin suppositories which can be given to the community for the initial treatment of severe malaria before transfer to a treatment centre.

A major obstacle to the large-scale use of artemisinin-based combination treatments has been their cost; they are up to ten times more expensive than chloroquine and other monotherapy schemes, and it has been difficult to see how these effective treatments would reach poor populations unless subsidies were introduced. The decision in 2001 to encourage most African countries to simultaneously change to artemisinin-based combination treatments, irrespective of their immediate need, contributed to a short-term quadrupling in the cost of artemisinin and a global shortage of raw materials, which was only overcome in the mid-2000s. Now, virtually every malaria-endemic country has adopted artemisinin-based combination treatments as the first line treatment but the proportion of children with malaria receiving these drugs remains low. There is recognition that widespread access to antimalarial drugs will only be achieved if costs for the patients are low. This has prompted a number of innovative initiatives being tried including by the 'Affordable Medicines Facility – malaria (AMF-m)' mechanism, which provides a subsidy that reduces the wholesale price of artemisinin-based combination treatments to a few cents. Linked to this expanded access to the most effective treatment for malaria when it is needed is the aim to reduce presumptive and unnecessary treatment of malaria by extending the use of rapid diagnostic tests for parasite diagnosis. Another major problem that needs to be addressed in many countries is the distribution of counterfeit sub-standard drugs.

The problem of having to re-treat bed nets with insecticides has been overcome by the development of long-lasting insecticidal nets, in which insecticide is incorporated into the net fibres. Inevitably, resistance to the recommended insecticides, the so-called pyrethroids, is emerging, but progress is being made towards identifying alternative insecticides to treat nets and other materials such as curtains that might be more acceptable in hot climates. Full cost recovery for nets, curtains and insecticides continue to make them unavailable to the most vulnerable and poorest people. Partial cost recovery by the use of vouchers, often combined with social marketing, has solved the problem to some extent. The preferred option of the free provision of insecticide treated nets, possibly linked to other initiatives such as routine vaccination of children or attendance at antenatal clinics, has gained momentum; although this approach requires a significant and sustained commitment from international donors.

Research in malaria-endemic areas has shown that giving antimalarial drugs during pregnancy at regular intervals to prevent malaria infections reduces the incidence of severe maternal anaemia and improves birthweight. Similarly, in young children, intermittent preventive treatment with antimalaria drugs lowers the incidence of malaria and severe anaemia. There is more research work to be done, but intermittent preventative treatment is a promising additional tool in malaria control. There has also been progress in malaria vaccine research over the past five to ten years, helped by the availability of more funds including from a major new player, the Bill and Melinda Gates Foundation, public–private partnerships in which major pharmaceutical companies participate and improved association mediated through organizations such as the Malaria Vaccine Initiative.

Malaria and poverty

Malaria and poverty are intimately connected, albeit not at the individual level: malaria does not discriminate between rich and poor victims. But malaria is particularly a problem in countries in the poorest continent, Africa. The only parts of Africa free of malaria are the northern and southern extremes, which have the richest countries of the continent. India, the country with the greatest number of poor people in the world, has a serious malaria problem. Haiti has the highest malaria mortality in the western hemisphere, and is the poorest country in the hemisphere. Malaria is geographically specific, as shown in

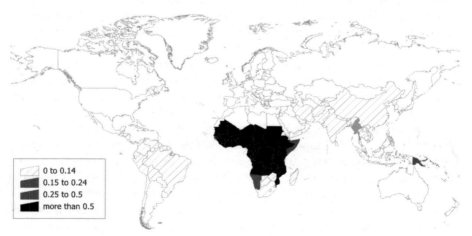

0 to 0.14
0.15 to 0.24
0.25 to 0.5
more than 0.5

Figure 2.2 *Map showing the global distribution of malaria risk (per 1000 population per year)*

Source: World Malaria Report 2008, World Health Organisation, Geneva, Switzerland, 2008.

Figure 2.2. The most intensive malaria problem is confined to the tropical world. Poverty is also geographically specific. As shown in Figure 2.3, poor countries predominate in regions where malaria is prevalent. Almost all of the rich countries are outside the bounds of intensive malaria.

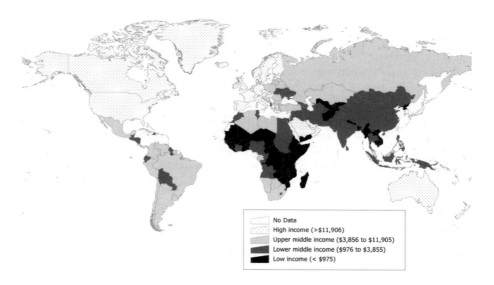

Figure 2.3 *Map showing the global distribution of income per capita*

Source: World Bank at www.worldbank.org (accessed on 24 February 2010)

Not only are malarial countries poor, economic growth in malarial countries is poor as well. Macroeconomist Jeffrey Sachs showed that growth of income per capita during the period 1965–1990 for countries with severe malaria was 0.4 per cent per year, whereas the average growth for other countries had been 2.3 per cent, or more than 5 times higher. The question then is whether malaria contributes to poverty and low growth, or does poverty cause higher malaria incidence, or is it both?

Poverty exacerbates malaria because poor households and governments do not have the financial means to fight the disease. Richer households can afford insecticide treated bed nets, they can afford to install screen doors and windows to help keep mosquitoes from entering the house in the first place, and they can ensure access to health care and effective medication when the need arises. It is estimated that 58 per cent of malaria deaths occur in the poorest 20 per cent of the world's population – a higher percentage than for any other disease of major public health importance.

But malaria also causes poverty. As we have seen, children who have malaria can suffer long-lasting ill effects. And with frequent disease episodes, they may drop out of school early because of poor attendance and a poor ability to learn. And their parents experience lost productivity and income associated with malaria illness or death in the household. When children are expected to die in large numbers, parents overcompensate and have more children, with serious consequences. Too poor to invest in the education of all their children, the family might educate just one or two children, usually the elder sons. If children from poor families in malaria-endemic regions manage to survive, they often enter adulthood without the proper education they need to survive. This is particularly true for girls.

The presence of malaria in a community or country also hampers individual and national prosperity due to its influence on social and economic decisions. The risk of contracting malaria can deter investment and can affect decision-making in many ways that have a negative impact on economic growth and productivity. Some examples include a preference by individual farmers/households to plant subsistence crops rather than more labour-intensive cash crops because of malaria's impact on labour during the harvest season; an underdeveloped tourist industry due to the reluctance of travellers to visit malaria-endemic areas; and undeveloped markets due to traders' unwillingness to travel and invest in malaria-endemic areas.

What can be done?

Malaria control, elimination or eradication?

The establishment of an effective malaria control programme – for example, strengthened vector control with indoor residual spraying with insecticide combined with active case finding and treatment with artemisinin combination treatment has resulted in marked and sustained malaria control in KwaZulu-Natal, South Africa. Achieving similar results in other sub-Saharan African countries which, unlike South Africa, suffer from an inadequate health infrastructure and high malaria-transmission rates seemed doubtful until recently and will certainly require sustained investment in health care delivery as well as subsidies for new drugs and other measures. Recent evidence that a similar impact can be achieved comes from highly-malaria endemic Zanzibar, where artemisinin combination treatment of diagnosed cases combined with the free distribution of long-lasting insecticidal bed nets has resulted in a dramatic reduction in the rates of malaria-related illness and deaths, and a ten-fold reduction of asymptomatic people having malaria parasites in their blood. This occurred shortly after the start of the programme, and while climatic conditions favourable for malaria transmission persisted during the observation period. In addition, there are reports of falling malaria illness and deaths in several other countries related to this strategy – in Asia (this is well-documented for Vietnam especially) and in eastern and southern Africa including Eritrea, Kenya, the mainland of Tanzania, Rwanda, Zambia and Mozambique, as well as west Africa including Senegal, Guinea Bissau and The Gambia (including the Farafenni area where Lamin lived). This relates to increased funding for malaria by governments and donor agencies. As a result some previously highly-endemic malaria countries are putting forward strategies to eliminate malaria. For example, Botswana, Namibia, South Africa and Swaziland have a 2015 elimination goal and they form a group with their northern neighbours Angola, Mozambique, Zambia and Zimbabwe (the last three were high transmission countries) where elimination is also planned, albeit at a slower pace.

Today, we are witnessing a redoubling of efforts and resources to attack the malaria problem, and this time the emphasis is on Africa, where the burden of malaria is greatest. The new efforts and resources are coming from governments and donor agencies such as the Bill and Melinda Gates Foundation, the (US) President's Malaria Initiative, the World Bank's booster programme and the Global Fund to fight AIDS, Tuberculosis and Malaria. The Global Fund that was created in 2002 to finance a dramatic turn-around in these three diseases, is claiming that up to November 2009 it helped by distributing 104 million insecticide treated bed nets, and delivered 108 million artemisinin-based combination drug treatments. Annual support for malaria control from international donors has now reached about US$1 billion a year. This is not enough to provide a comprehensive global control programme, estimated to require about $5 billion a year, but it is a major step forward and has allowed the widespread deployment of insecticide treated bed nets and artemisinin-based combination treatments in many malaria endemic countries. Indoor spraying with residual insecticides using pyrethroids or DDT is also being used (again) on an increasing scale. Scaling-up and getting things done in-country remains one of the major challenges, and strengthening the health systems in many countries will have to go hand in hand with supporting the specific efforts to tackle malaria.

The international community continues to face difficult decisions about how to balance efforts in discovery, development and implementation of new tools against malaria. Malaria elimination in defined geographical areas, especially on the fringes of areas with high malaria transmission, might be achievable, but existing tools are insufficient to meet the ambitious tool of global eradication. New concepts and tools will be required to achieve eradication, including a necessity to pursue vaccine-development and new anti-vector measures, as well as new drugs.

The unexpected degree of success of the widespread deployment of effective treatment and vector control programmes in reducing the clinical burden of malaria in many countries has raised the bar for malaria vaccines whose target is primarily the prevention of disease (aimed at the pre-erythrocytic stage, providing a level of protection that prevents invasion of the blood and hence any clinical malaria). Vaccines with 30 per cent efficacy that persists for one to two years, which might have been deployed a few years ago, no longer have a useful role in combating malaria. A much higher level of efficacy will be required if malaria vaccines of this kind are to have a major role in future malaria control or elimination programmes. It is widely accepted that existing control tools will not be sufficient to interrupt transmission in areas where this occurs at a high level. Drugs that target the sexual stage of the parasite provide a possible tool for use in the final stages of an elimination programme but as the drug or drug combination must be given to the whole population, it must be extremely safe and no such drug currently exists. An alternative approach, but with the same criteria of having to be given to the whole population and therefore requiring high safety, is a vaccine that interrupts transmission. Vaccines with transmission-blocking potential (at the sporozoite or gametocyte stages) are being developed, and are likely to become an increasingly important objective of malaria vaccine development programmes. Transmission-blocking vaccines could prove to be especially important in aiding the elimination of *Plasmodium vivax*, the dominant parasite in Asia. *P. vivax* presents special problems as it has dormant stages in the liver (hypnozoites) that can persist for months or years, periodically giving rise to relapse infections; this makes it more difficult to eliminate *P. vivax* than *P. falciparum*.

As Brian Greenwood (*Journal of Clinical Investigation*), one of the world's leading malariologists, and godfather of many of the current generation of malaria scientists, and others have recently argued, the future success of malaria control, elimination and eradication efforts will depend 'on how well the scientific and public health communities can work together to extend the effective life span of our existing tools while discerning new interventions that interrupt the complex life cycle of *Plasmodium* parasites.' The prevention and treatment of malaria is possible. At a cost of about $5 per person per year it is possible to establish an effective malaria control programme, for example, one centred around insecticide treated bed nets or indoor residual spraying for prevention and artemisinin combination therapy for treatment. This sounds like a small amount of money, but it also represents a week's wages for many average-sized families in poor countries. Wide coverage can be obtained with these simple interventions, but subsidies will be needed for the poor. It is important that the international community sustains and even increases its support for the initiative of the Global Fund against AIDS, Tuberculosis, and Malaria and other agencies dedicated to increasing access to these tools. Lamin, and many others, have died unnecessarily from malaria, and many others will, but let's make certain that the numbers continue to decrease – it is possible.

Sources and suggestions for further reading

For the history of malaria, Desowitz's *The Malaria Capers. Tales of People and Parasites* (W. W. Norton & Company, 1991, New York) and S. Litsios's *The Tomorrow of Malaria* (Pacific Press, Wellington, New Zealand, 2nd edition, 1997) are both highly readable and informative and also contain quotes from Walpole, Laveran and Manson that can be found on pages 151, 167 and 35.

Essential Malariology (David Warrell and Herbert Gilles, published by Arnold, 2002) is the standard textbook that covers the clinical, laboratory and public health aspects of malaria, and is also a practical guide for all who are involved in the diagnosis, treatment and prevention of the disease. Excellent recent review papers on malaria include Brian Greenwood et al., 'Malaria' that was published in *The Lancet* (2005; 365: 1487--1498), and Brian Greenwood et al., 'Malaria: progress, perils, and prospects for eradication' in the *Journal of Clinical Investigation* (2008; 118: 1266–1276), and Brian Greenwood and Geoffrey Targett, 'Do we still need a malaria vaccine? *Parasite Immunology* (2009; 31: 582–586). The 'averting a malaria paper' by Nick White and colleagues was published in *The Lancet* in 1999; 353: 1965–1967. Jeffrey Sachs's *The End of Poverty* (Penguin, New York, 2007) is one of three books with very different ideas on how to tackle world poverty that I refer to in this book (the other ones being Paul Collier's *The Bottom Billion* (see Chapter 12) and William Easterly's *The White Man's Burden* (see Chapter 1)). *Shrinking the Malaria Map. A Prospectus on Malaria Elimination* (edited by Richard Feacham, Allison Phillips and Geoffrey Targett; The Global Health Group, Global Health Sciences, University of California, San Francisco, 2009) is a detailed and practical road map, providing direction and options including tools from which to choose a path towards malaria elimination. The paper by Achuyt Bhattarai and others entitled 'Impact of artemisinin-based combination therapy and insecticide-treated nets on malaria burden on Zanzibar' in *PLoS Medicine* (2007; 4: e309), strongly suggests that artemisinin-based combination therapy together with the widespread use of long-lasting impregnated nets could help achieve the goal of eliminating malaria even in moderate to highly malaria endemic countries. Indices of falling malaria illness and deaths in The Gambia were reported in *The Lancet* by Serign Ceesay and colleagues in 2008 (372: 1545–1554). A. Kameko et al. (*The Lancet* 2000; 356: 1560–1564) describes malaria elimination from a range of islands, including Taiwan and Mauritius. The text of the Stockholm Convention on Persistent Organic Pollutants can be found at the website www.chm.pops.

3
TB and HIV

If disease is an expression of individual life under unfavourable conditions, then epidemics must be indicators of mass disturbances in mass life.

Rudolf Virchow, 1848

Ramesh

If you travel the highway from Mumbai airport in the direction of the city centre, you can catch a glimpse of Juhu, one of the largest slums in the world. Juhu is not dissimilar to Garib Nagar, the Mumbai slum famous as the location of the eight-Oscars award winning movie *Slumdog Millionaire*. In Juhu lives Ramesh, 22 years old, with his parents, his two younger brothers and one sister in a two room shack. Until he became too sick to work, Ramesh was the single breadwinner of the family, earning US$2 per day as a shop assistant in a near-by corner shop. That Ramesh did not seek health care early was a combination of having to deal with the illness of his father who had recently had a stroke, the family's dire financial situation, and a failure to realize the severity of his condition. Ramesh had, when he went to see a doctor, all the classic signs and symptoms of lung tuberculosis: severe productive cough – sometimes blood stained – for more than one month, night fevers and weight loss of more than 10kg. His chest X-ray confirmed the abnormal findings that the doctor found on auscultation, with a large lesion in the upper and middle lobe of the right lung. His sputum contained acid-fast bacilli (diagnostic for tuberculosis, later confirmed by culture). He was also severely wasted, anaemic and had a generalized skin rash. He agreed to have an HIV test after counselling: the initial test plus a confirmatory test were both positive for HIV. Ramesh's CD4 cell count, a measure of the number of disease-fighting cells in the blood, was at a low level of 200 cells per mm³. Ramesh was admitted to hospital and standard multi-drug treatments for TB, and later for AIDS, were started, as well as symptomatic treatment for the anaemia and skin rash.

Tuberculosis

Germany is in terrible condition this year. This is particularly true of the working classes, who are so undernourished that tuberculosis is having a rich harvest, particularly of adolescent children

Agnes Medley, 1921

Tuberculosis has troubled mankind throughout history. Spread through the air from one person to another when an infected person coughs or sneezes, the bacteria that cause tuberculosis usually attack the lungs. However, tuberculosis can attack other parts of the body, including the kidneys, the spine and the brain. Evidence of tuberculosis appears in Chinese literature dating back to around 4000 BC, and in religious books in India to around 2000 BC. In ancient Greece around 400 BC, Hippocrates mentions tuberculosis, as does Aristotle, who talked about 'phthisis' (from the Greek word to waste away). The 'great white plague' which started in Europe in the 1600s and continued for more than 200 years was tuberculosis. Other commonly used names throughout history for tuberculosis besides phthisis and the white plague, are scrofula (swellings of the lymph nodes of the neck), consumption (progressive wasting away of the body), and TB (the presence or products of the tubercle bacillus). Dying of tuberculosis was especially common among young, poor people but the elite did not escape from the disease. Tuberculosis cut short the life of such cultural icons as John Keats, Frederyk Chopin, Franz Kafka and George Orwell. Although often fatal, tuberculosis tended to be romanticized in the 19th century, as can be seen in the figure of Violetta in Verdi's opera *La Traviata*, first staged in Venice in 1853. At that time, tuberculosis was considered a disorder of people predisposed through heredity. Generations of languishing, beautiful women were not considered infectious, but only glamorously frail, their short lives akin to the beauty of moths fluttering around a candle flame.

Robert Koch (1843–1910) can be regarded as the godfather of bacteriology, and his methodology for the detection of acid-fast bacilli on microscopic examination, remains the gold standard for the bacteriological diagnosis of tuberculosis. Koch announced his discovery of the organism that causes tuberculosis, *Mycobacterium tuberculosis*, in March 1882 at a meeting of the Berlin Physiological Society. By 1896, when Puccini's opera *La Bohème* was staged for the first time in Turin, Puccini and the world knew that tuberculosis was an infectious disease, aggravated by the cramped, dirty conditions of the poor. Mimi is still as beautiful and as tragically doomed as Violetta, but the setting in *La Bohème* is much more socially realistic and scientifically true than in *La Traviata*. There is much in the opera about Mimi's racking cough and what it means, and her lover, the poet Rodolfo, casts her off because he fears the implications of her illness.

The news of Koch's work on the discovery of the tuberculosis bacillus caused enormous excitement throughout the world and was summarized by scientists in letters in the London *Times* and later in the *New York Times*. Not unreasonably, editorial writers assumed that Koch's discovery would lead to a treatment for tuberculosis. People wanted to believe that this would happen; for centuries tuberculosis had been feared as the 'captain of the men of death', and in the 19th century it caused about one in every seven deaths in Europe and the Americas. It was not surprising, therefore, that the news of Koch's discovery raised unrealistic hopes for its immediate control. In fact it took over 60 years before an effective treatment became available. The medical measures available to control tuberculosis remained modest, but improving social and sanitary conditions and ensuring adequate nutrition reduced the inter-personal spread of disease and strengthened the body's defences against the tuberculosis bacillus. Thousands of sanatoria were established throughout Europe and the Americas, providing a dual function: isolating the sick, and thus the source of infection, from the general population, while forced rest in fresh air, together with a proper diet and a well-regulated hospital life assisted the healing processes.

In 1944 Selman Waksman, a Russian who had migrated to the US, announced the discovery of an antibiotic produced by the soil organism *Streptomyces griseus*, which he called streptomycin. It turned out that this agent was active against tuberculosis. Use of streptomycin alone rapidly led, however, to resistant strains and it was found more effective in combination in the so-called 'triple-therapy' with para-amino-salicylic acid (introduced in 1949) and isonic-otinic acid hydrazide, or isoniazid (1952). Other antituberculosis drugs followed, including pyrazinamide (1954), cycloserine (1955), ethambutol (1962) and rifampicin (1963). Long-term combination therapy became the norm in tuberculosis treatment.

In 1900, in the US, tuberculosis was responsible for 110 deaths per 100,000 people per year, by 1950 it had fallen to 22; by 1960, when several different antituberculosis drugs were available, it was 5.4; in 1975 it was 1.2. We will never know whether the prevalence of the disease would have continued to decline as it did even if the antituberculosis drugs had not been discovered, but their availability certainly had an enormous impact on clinical practice in the 1950s. Within a few years most sanatoria in rich countries had either been dismantled or converted to 'chest hospitals', in which were treated diseases that replaced tuberculosis as the bread and butter of chest physicians – chronic bronchitis, emphysema and lung cancer, for example.

Not long ago many experts thought that tuberculosis would be controlled by antibiotics, but that has changed. The most recent estimates of the world epidemic of tuberculosis are for 2007, when there were 9.3 million new cases and 1.7 million deaths. Figure 3.1 shows that the high burden of new cases is mainly in African, Asian and former Soviet Union countries. Half of the new cases were in Asia (with 2.0 million new cases in India alone) and a third in Africa. Tuberculosis has enormous economic consequences as more than 80 per cent of cases are among working people aged between 15 and 65. The limitations of existing methods for the prevention, diagnosis and treatment of tuberculosis have been emphasized by the increased susceptibility of HIV-infected people to develop the disease, and the emergence of strains resistant to combination drug-therapy. In 1993 the World Health Organization declared tuberculosis an international health emergency.

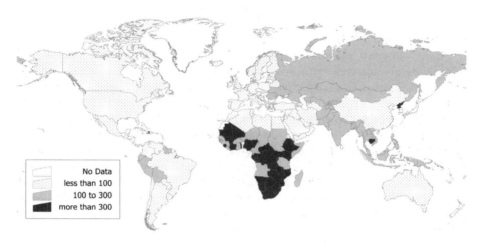

Figure 3.1 *Map showing the global distribution of new cases of tuberculosis (per 100,000 population per year)*

Source: *Millenium Development Goals Indicators*. The official United Nations site for the MDG indicators at mdgs.un.org/unsd/mdg (accessed on 17 February 2010)

Microscopy is still the cornerstone of the diagnosis of lung tuberculosis, 125 years after its discovery. The method is attractive because the relatively simple equipment required has other uses and, in settings with a high prevalence of tuberculosis, microscopy is specific for the diagnosis. However, bacteria must be present in high concentrations in the sputum to be detected, and HIV-infected patients often have a low bacterial burden, which reduces the sensitivity of microscopy where HIV is prevalent. A very disturbing fact is that probably more than half of the cases of sputum-positive tuberculosis remain undetected. In regions of the world where microscopy has the poorest performance, the need for early detection of tuberculosis is the greatest. Better access to diagnostic services and education of health professionals, and via them of patients, along with providing simple but good sputum-submission guidance, might increase the number of patients being examined while also substantially increasing the detection of tuberculosis.

Conventional 'short-course' therapy for tuberculosis has remained unchanged for decades. The most frequently recommended and effective combination is isoniazid, rifampicin, pyrazinamide and ethambutol for two months, followed by isoniazid and rifampicin for another four months. Under practical programme conditions, completion rates of therapy are variable, partly because many patients find it difficult to continue with their daily treatment once their symptoms improve. Failure to complete therapy is associated with remaining infectious, relapse and drug resistance. Directly Observed Therapy, Short course (DOTS) involves the supervision of every dose of tuberculosis medication for six months by clinic staff, community health workers or family members in an attempt to improve treatment completion. The search is on for new antituberculosis drugs to improve treatment for patients with multi-drug resistant tuberculosis, and to enable the treatment to be shortened.

It is estimated that more than 4 per cent of patients with tuberculosis worldwide are infected with a multi-drug resistant strain, and treatment for this is prolonged, less effective, costly and poorly tolerated. Even more alarming, a considerable and increasing proportion of multi-drug resistant tuberculosis cases are caused by what is called 'extensively drug-resistant tuberculosis'. This terminology doesn't do justice to the seriousness of this condition, as it describes a level of resistance that makes tuberculosis extremely difficult to treat with the current arsenal of drugs available. During the time that Ramesh was receiving his treatment for tuberculosis, the hospital director's daughter died from drug-resistant tuberculosis. She had been working as a doctor on an infectious diseases ward in another Mumbai hospital, got a headache and low-grade fevers, started vomiting, became confused and developed neck stiffness. Analysis of the cerebrospinal fluid revealed that she had tuberculous meningitis. She was treated with standard treatment and other drugs were added when tests revealed multi-drug resistant tuberculosis. Despite this she died after two months of treatment.

Another problem is smear-negative disease, which cannot be detected with microscopy. Although such disease has a lower transmission potential, it contributes importantly to global tuberculosis disease and mortality. Launched at the World Health Assembly in 2003, with initial funding from the Bill and Melinda Gates Foundation, the Foundation for Innovative New Diagnostics is working with industry and academic groups to replace or improve microscopy with appropriate technologies for the level of the health system at which they would be used to detect smear-positive tuberculosis. Work is also ongoing to develop new diagnostic tools for case detection for smear-negative disease, drug susceptibility testing and for the detection of latent infection. Technologies are being developed for different levels of the health care system to match the human resources available and the degree of complexity of the diagnostic question, with a prioritization of those tests that can be used at the most peripheral level where most patients first seek care.

The Bacillus Calmette-Guérin (BCG) vaccine, created at the Pasteur Institute in Paris in 1921, is the only existing vaccine against tuberculosis. It is prepared from a strain of the attenuated (weakened) live bovine tuberculosis bacillus, *Mycobacterium bovis*, which has lost its virulence in humans by being specially cultured in an artificial medium for years. It provides some protection against severe forms of tuberculosis in children, such as meningitis, but is unreliable against adult lung tuberculosis especially in tropical poor countries.

Because it protects children, the World Health Organization recommends that BCG is given to all children born in countries highly endemic for tuberculosis.

In recent years, a number of new vaccine candidates for tuberculosis have been developed and have shown promising results when tested in animals. A few of them are entering human safety trials. Some of these vaccines are designed to over-express certain tuberculosis antigens that are recognized by the immune system, thereby preparing the body's defences for exposure to *Mycobacterium tuberculosis*. Other candidate vaccines aim to prevent the bacteria from hiding in cells (hiding is the strategy by which the bacteria evades the body's immune system). New tuberculosis vaccines to prevent childhood and adult forms of tuberculosis, to prevent progression of latent tuberculosis to the active disease stage (it is estimated that one-third of the world population is infected with the tubercle bacilli), and to shorten drug treatment regimens or reduce the risk of relapse, could fundamentally alter our approach to tuberculosis control.

But while we await new diagnostics, drugs and vaccines, a pressing need to address a tuberculosis catastrophe exists: the HIV-driven epidemic, especially in sub-Saharan Africa. Of the 9.3 million reported incident cases of tuberculosis in 2007, 1.3 million were co-infected with HIV. As many as 456,000 co-infected individuals died, making tuberculosis the most common cause of death in people with HIV. Despite the difficulties described above, tuberculosis is still a preventable and treatable disease, but thrives amid weak health systems. Attitudes to tuberculosis will have to change among health professionals and the public. Laboratories and clinicians need to follow best practice in diagnosis, reporting and managing the disease – and they need the tools to do so. Additionally, efforts to control tuberculosis should engage communities to reduce stigma, support care and develop local solutions. These are not so different from the control programmes needed for tuberculosis' terrible twin: HIV.

HIV

Every day, almost three times as many people become newly infected with HIV as those who start taking antiretroviral treatment. We will set ourselves up for demoralization and failure if we base our strategies on the illusion that the end of AIDS can be achieved any time soon.

Peter Piot, 2008

On 5 June 1981 the US Centers for Disease Control and Prevention (CDC) reported five cases of immune-deficiency disease with pneumonia caused by *Pneumocystis carinii* in gay men living in Los Angeles. Although the CDC first believed that the new disease was confined to homosexual men, by the end of the year cases had been reported in non-homosexual injecting drug users and outside the US (in the UK). Other immune-deficiency diseases were soon reported in different populations from many countries, including Haiti and some African countries. In May 1983, a retrovirus (which was later termed the human immunodeficiency virus, or HIV) was isolated from a patient with AIDS in France by Luc Montagnier and Françoise Barré-Sinoussi, at the Pasteur Institute in Paris. Around 22 months later, the US Food and Drug Administration approved a commercial test to detect the virus. By 1985, over 17,000 cases of AIDS from 71 countries had been reported to the World Health Organization in Geneva.

Through much of the 1980s, it seemed almost incomprehensible to most policy-makers and the public at large that overlapping sexual and needle-sharing networks had somehow led to tens of thousands of people around the world being infected with HIV. The disease seemed to be concentrated in marginalized populations. Many governments denied that HIV or its associated risk behaviours existed in their countries. A few epidemiologists and activists began to project that the epidemic would become a worldwide pandemic that would outstrip tuberculosis. For the most part they met widespread scepticism. At the same time, the epidemic started to get media attention, in part because it also affected well-known figures, including the son of Zambia's president Kenneth Kaunda, UK rock band Queen's Freddy Mercury and the Ugandan pop star Philly Lutaaya, the French philosopher Michel Foucault, and American celebrities like the actor Rock Hudson and the basketball star Magic Johnson.

The brief media flurry of the late 1980s and early 1990s soon faded, but the virus spread relentlessly around the world during the 1990s. By the late 1990s, HIV prevalence was slightly less than 1 per cent globally and averaged 6 per cent in sub-Saharan Africa amongst adults aged 15–49. Although information on how HIV is transmitted was known early in the pandemic, the initial response to the disease was delayed, grossly insufficient, fragmented and inconsistent. As white homosexuals accounted for the vast majority of AIDS cases in the US in the mid-1980s, the characterization of the disease as a gay disease created a strong worldwide stigma that was fed by existing moral beliefs and prejudice about gay sex in many countries, including those in Africa and the Caribbean, where the pandemic was smouldering. The widely circulating photos of wasted patients with AIDS in Africa dying from 'slim disease', for which there was no cure, created a climate of fear and fuelled the mounting discrimination and denial about the disease. Many religious organizations, while compassionately caring for patients with AIDS, refused to promote condoms or provide sexual education to youths because they perceived this as condoning or encouraging promiscuity.

Since the end of the 1990s HIV prevalence has stabilized globally with treatment becoming available more widely, although the absolute number of people living with HIV/AIDS continues to increase in line with population growth. There are now an estimated 33 million people living with HIV. In 2007 there were 2.5 million new infections, and 2.1 million people died from AIDS related illnesses. A quarter of a century into the pandemic, with no vaccine in sight and the number of new infections still outpacing the progress in access to treatment, we clearly need to take a long-term view in planning our actions.

Research in the 1980s determined the precise means by which HIV invades the body. Transmitted from person to person primarily through semen, vaginal secretions and blood, HIV's principal targets are cells of the immune system (the 'disease fighting' CD4 cells/macrophages) which are intended to clear foreign pathogens from the body. After entering a cell of the immune system, the virus begins a relentless process of replication, its sole activity and one that allows for a constant spread to new cells. In the process, the immune system can be devastated. The HIV life cycle requires the insertion of its own genetic material into the host cell and the use of three important viral enzymes. These three enzymes are essential to the process of viral replication, and most advances in HIV treatment have come from inhibiting the activity of these enzymes.

In 1986 the US Food and Drug Administration approved the first antiviral drug zidovudine ('AZT') for use in preventing HIV replication. Between 1986 and 1991 the standard antiviral therapy for HIV-infected individuals who had access to these, at the time, very expensive drugs was 'monotherapy': treatment with a single drug. As with tuberculosis, treatment of HIV with a single drug rapidly led to resistance. The discovery of a number of distinct classes of antiviral medications made it possible to shift from monotherapy to combination therapy, in which drugs from two or more classes of antivirals with different actions were used simultaneously. These drug combinations are referred to as 'highly active antiretroviral therapy' or HAART. The news about the effectiveness of combination therapy broke in 1996, at that year's International AIDS conference in Vancouver. Following the conference, a spate of news coverage suggested an end to the AIDS epidemic. The *New York Times Magazine* headline 'When plagues end: notes on the twilight of an epidemic' gave false hope, especially to hundreds of thousands of poor people without any possibility of accessing the unaffordable treatment, and was misleading. Combination therapy was not and is not, a miracle cure as it does not eliminate HIV from the body, which means that people need to continue their strict schedule of medications (that have unpleasant side effects) lifelong.

I first encountered HIV in 1983 when I had my initial experience with health care in poor countries as a medical intern, working for a four-month period in a rural hospital in northwest Tanzania. At that time, I and my much more experienced senior colleagues did not recognize that the case of Kaposi's sarcoma we were treating was associated with HIV. In the next 20 years as a physician working mostly in rural East and West Africa, I treated several hundreds of HIV-positive people, some of whom were colleagues and friends. I have had to watch most of them die an early and slow, painful death. In 2002, a friend and colleague in Farafenni, The Gambia, was found to be very sick with HIV-related illnesses. He was to become the first person I had met in rural Africa who was able to access antiretroviral treatment. He had to travel monthly for his medication to a government clinic in Kaolack in neighbouring Senegal, which had just started a treatment programme with support from the Global Fund against AIDS, Malaria and Tuberculosis. He is still on daily treatment today, and well.

In 2003 the World Health Organization declared poor access to antiretroviral medicines as another international health emergency. The organization led by its then Director-General Lee Jong-wook spearheaded an initiative with the 'three by five' target: provision of treatment to three million people in poor countries by the end of 2005. Around the same time – the end 2003/early 2004, the William [Bill] J. Clinton Foundation brokered agreements with 'Big Pharma', as well as leading medical technology companies, to launch two major price-reduction agreements. The two agreements reduced the costs of testing for and treating HIV/AIDS from $3600 to around $250 per patient per year in poor countries. Although the goal of three million people – out of an estimated need for therapy of 9.7 million people – was not reached until the end of 2007, 'three by five' played an important role in catalysing action to expand treatment access in poor countries.

Unfortunately, the access to medicines campaign was not matched by an access to prevention campaign. Only 20 per cent of people with HIV in poor countries are aware of their HIV status. Surveys indicate that only 40 per cent of men and 38 per cent of women aged 15–24 years have accurate and comprehensive knowledge about HIV and how to avoid transmission. Once again, policy-makers failed to achieve the right balance between prevention and treatment efforts early on in the epidemic by largely ignoring care and support needs in poor countries, and more recently by investing in a rapid and urgently needed expansion of antiretroviral treatment without simultaneously expanding prevention efforts.

In February 2004, Richard Holbrooke, then President of the Global Business Coalition on HIV/AIDS, made a plea in the *New York Times* for routine testing for HIV. He made the case that testing should be routine at marriage, before childbirth and at any visit to a hospital. Holbrooke argued that widespread or routine testing for HIV is an important method of preventing the spread of HIV. He felt that testing was not given a high priority because of a locked mindset from the time when stigmatization was a much larger problem and when antiretroviral treatment was unavailable.

AIDS, sex and drugs

> *The World Bank believes poverty and gender inequality spread AIDS. I believe sex and drug injection spread AIDS.*
>
> Elizabeth Pisani, 2008

And I believe it is all of the above that spread AIDS, while I am also convinced that there are large differences between populations in the relative importance of factors. HIV is spread in a very heterogeneous way worldwide, and even within countries the risk of contracting HIV varies widely. Often there is a mismatch between the populations at greatest risk of becoming infected or transmitting HIV and efforts to reach them with prevention activities. A very important barrier in many countries is not lack of knowledge about which populations should be targeted, but rather the political, legal, cultural or social barriers that hinder the implementation of targeted plans. Contextual factors, determinants of risk factors and barriers to prevention are of greatest importance in planning intervention programmes. Most new HIV infections in adolescents and adults are transmitted via sexual intercourse, and to a lesser extent through the sharing of needles among injecting drug users. Abstinence, having safe sexual intercourse or having unsafe sexual intercourse is often but not always an individual decision, and that decision is clearly affected by peers, family, community and context.

There is no vaccine against HIV, and the difficulties and surprises that the search for an HIV vaccine have experienced over the past 25 years with an estimated investment of more than $1 billion, make it a risky business to predict when an effective vaccine might become available. Traditional approaches have failed. While vaccines for infections such as polio are designed to stimulate the body to produce antibodies, this approach has failed in HIV vaccine research, as variability in the virus's structure, both within and between patients, has resulted in responses to vaccines being too narrow and too weak. Difficulties in HIV vaccine research include the properties of the virus in that HIV damages the very immune cells that are needed for an effective vaccine response, and that HIV is genetically diverse with three main groups containing distinct clades that are found in different proportions across the globe. In addition, HIV converts its genetic material from ribonucleic acid (RNA) into DNA after it infects cells, before hiding this DNA away within the human CD4 cells, ready to start producing more HIV particles at any time. This means that an effective HIV vaccine must be able to stimulate a long-lasting immune response to prevent HIV production within the body. And lastly, vaccines that were designed to target proteins on the surface of the HIV particle were ineffective as it is now understood that these proteins change shape and position when they bind to receptors on the surface of an antibody cell. Most experts predict that no vaccine will be available for at least another 20 years.

The male condom, if used correctly and consistently, has proven to be effective in blocking HIV transmission during sexual intercourse. The problem is that the use of male condoms depends on the willingness of men to use them. In areas of the world most greatly affected by HIV, women and young girls account for most of those infected. Socio-cultural, economic and gender-inequality differentials contribute to the high incidence of HIV among women who are restricted in their ability to negotiate the use of male condoms. Female-initiated methods, including physical barriers (female condom, cervical diaphragm) and topical antimicrobial (microbicide) products, will need to be easy to use, cheap, non-toxic and effective in the prevention of HIV transmission during sexual intercourse. So far they are not.

Hardly related to sex and drugs, and much more to poverty and gender inequality, are the children under the age of 15 who became infected with HIV (around 430,000 in 2008 alone), mainly though mother-to-child transmission (MTCT). About 80 per cent of these MTCT infections occurred in Africa where in several countries AIDS is beginning to reverse several decades of progress in child survival. MTCT is when an HIV-infected woman passes the virus to her baby, and this can occur during pregnancy, labour and delivery, or breastfeeding. Without treatment, around 15–30 per cent of infants born to HIV positive mothers will become infected with HIV during pregnancy and delivery, while a further 5–20 per cent will become infected through breastfeeding. In rich countries, MTCT has been reduced to less than 2 per cent thanks to effective voluntary testing and counselling, access to antiretroviral therapy, safe delivery practices including elective caesarean section and the widespread availability and safe use of breast-milk substitutes. If these interventions were used in poor countries as well, they could save the lives of thousands of children each year. Unfortunately, in many poor country settings, elective caesarean sections and avoidance of breastfeeding are often unsafe, unacceptable and unaffordable. In addition, providing basic antiretroviral therapy for mother and infant in the period around delivery is not being achieved. There is an urgent need to scale up the prevention and treatment of HIV infections in children, focusing on strengthening prevention of mother-to-child transmission programmes in order to reduce the number of infants who are infected in addition to reducing morbidity and mortality among their mothers.

As no one-dimensional biomedical HIV/AIDS solution is available, 'combination prevention' is as necessary as 'combination treatment' when it comes to stopping the pandemic. Epidemiological modelling suggests that even the most solidly proven cost-effective biomedical intervention which reduces HIV transmission — male circumcision – cannot be a 'stand-alone': an increase in risky sexual behaviour after circumcision could offset the beneficial effects of circumcision if not prevented by means of appropriate health education, including routine HIV testing. Effective HIV prevention also requires locally contextualized approaches that address both individual and social norms and structures, and are grounded in human rights. When one considers the elements of a prevention programme needed to reduce the incidence of HIV among gay men in Los Angeles, female sex workers in Mumbai (Ramesh believes he became HIV infected from unprotected sex with a female sex worker), injecting drug users in Dushanbe or discordant couples in Kampala, the diversity of approaches required becomes very apparent. There is a globally useful distinction between concentrated and generalized epidemics. Epidemics are *concentrated* if transmission occurs largely in defined vulnerable groups – typically men who have sex with men, sex workers or injecting drug users, and their partners – and if protecting them would protect wider society.

Conversely, epidemics are *generalized* if transmission is sustained by sexual behaviour in the general population and would persist despite effective programmes for vulnerable groups. With a broad brush stroke approach one can state that the epidemics in Southern and Eastern Africa are generalized (as also shown in Figure 3.2), while the ones in Asia, including India, are concentrated. Unfortunately between these extremes, it is less clear whether some epidemics in West and Central Africa are concentrated, low-grade generalized or mixed.

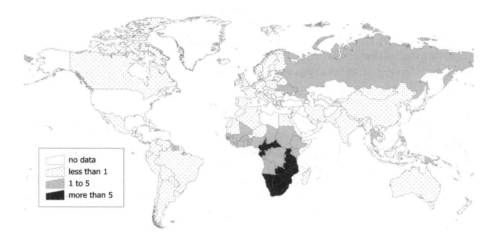

no data
less than 1
1 to 5
more than 5

Figure 3.2 *Map showing the global distribution of prevalence of HIV among population aged 15–49 (%)*

Source: *Millenium Development Goals Indicators.* The official United Nations site for the MDG indicators at mdgs.un.org/unsd/mdg (accessed on 17 February 2010)

Once we better understand our epidemics, can we respond with proven approaches? Where it is transmission in men who have sex with men that fuels HIV epidemics, the real-world picture is not very encouraging. However, there is greater room for optimism in contexts that are more open to homosexuality. If we face concentrated epidemics fuelled by sex work, we know what to do. Targeted interventions that promote education, condoms, sexual health, solidarity, empowerment and rights for sex workers have proven successful. And for injecting drug users there is again good evidence of what works: a comprehensive approach that includes clean needle and syringe programmes, opioid substitution therapy with, for example, methadone; condom programmes for users and their sexual partners; targeted information provision; sexually transmitted infections and tuberculosis prevention, diagnosis and treatment. Unfortunately, many countries and programmes are struggling to find the right balance between minimization of harm to injecting drug users with the goal of reducing the supply of and demand for illicit drugs.

There are often inconsistencies in policy and practice, and we have failed to convince the authorities in many countries that comprehensive harm reduction strategies are preferable to coercive approaches.

Lessons learned from the successes in reducing population-level HIV prevalence in countries such as Uganda with generalized epidemics may prove useful for prevention programming. In Uganda a mix of communication channels disseminated simple and clear messages about several risk reduction and health-seeking options including delaying first intercourse, a reduction in the number of partners, condom use especially with non-primary partners, HIV testing and treatment for sexually transmitted infections. It was important that one risk reduction strategy (e.g. abstinence or partner reduction) was not emphasized over another (e.g. condom use), thereby giving people a choice and contributing to the availability of a mix of strategies. Local involvement, with national government support, in message design, production and dissemination was another important feature.

However, one approach is applicable everywhere and an absolute must. Any sustainable effect on the future of HIV/AIDS will depend on the behaviour of young people, the adults of tomorrow. Even in those settings where the epidemic is still limited and concentrated in specific risk groups, we need to ensure that all young people, before they become sexually active, have the information they need to prevent infection with HIV, given that the epidemic is dynamic, changing and rarely stays in any one risk group. Age-appropriate universal sex education is clearly needed from primary-school age. Sex education has never been shown to encourage promiscuity, as is sometimes claimed. In fact, the weight of evidence shows that it encourages the delay of sexual activity and higher rates of protected sex.

What is also needed everywhere is good political leadership. Bad politics, including the absence of leadership, is one of the main obstacles to effective HIV prevention. 'Tied aid' allows a country or organization to avoid supporting something it doesn't like – such as condom use. HIV prevention requires addressing sex and drugs. In view of the associated political risks, policy-makers are naturally reluctant to advocate HIV prevention programmes that are larger than the programme scale demanded by the public. Thus, rather than leading the public, decision-makers often lag behind public opinion. Additionally, short political cycles bias public policy in favour of expenditures that will produce visible returns in the short term, and thus against prevention activities that produce their results in the medium to long term. Unfortunately, public policy often favours the treatment of infected individuals over disease prevention.

TB, HIV and poverty

> *Tuberculosis and HIV/AIDS cannot be dissociated. The co-infection must be tackled together. Collaborative tuberculosis/ HIV activities on a limited or sporadic basis are not enough.*
>
> Jorge Sampaio, 2007

Tuberculosis is the archetypal disease of poverty. Of the 22 countries that have 80 per cent of the world's tuberculosis disease burden, 17 are classified as low-income countries. Within these countries, the poorest have least access to treatment. Even in those countries with strong tuberculosis control programmes that offer free diagnosis and treatment, the poor can face catastrophic health expenditure because of the high costs of care before diagnosis, loss of income because of the disease and high indirect costs during treatment. The shortfall of $1.6 billion on a total amount of $4.6 billion needed for global tuberculosis control in 2009 can rightfully be called shameful, particularly when it is estimated that each dollar spent on care generates $15 in productivity.

Globally, the highest HIV prevalence rates are found in poor countries, but in sub-Saharan Africa, the poorest countries do not necessarily have the highest prevalence rates. Nevertheless, poverty increases vulnerability to HIV/AIDS and exacerbates the devastation of the epidemic. Poverty deprives people of the means to cope with HIV. The poor more often than the rich lack the knowledge, awareness, skills and power to enable them to protect themselves from the virus, and, once infected, they are less able to gain access to care and life-prolonging treatment. It is estimated that the total resources available for HIV/AIDS have grown from less than $300 million in 1996 to around $10 billion in 2007. Development assistance programmes such as the Global Fund against HIV/AIDS, Tuberculosis and Malaria, the US President's Emergency Plan for AIDS relief, and the World Bank's Africa multi-country AIDS programme have helped to channel assistance to the countries in most need. However, prevention spending has grown much less than spending for treatment. The mismatch between the populations at greatest risk of becoming infected or transmitting HIV and efforts made to reach them with prevention programmes is another concern.

Both tuberculosis and HIV/AIDS strike young adults in their most productive years, and they therefore have a particularly destructive effect on families and households and on the long-term economic development of a country. In societies where teachers and health professionals are dying as well as farmers and miners, HIV/AIDS and tuberculosis will make another generation poor unless the epidemics are controlled. This is best done in a coordinated and integrated manner. Ramesh responded well to standard multi-drug treatment for TB, and he was discharged from hospital after ten days. Now, ten months later, Ramesh has completed his six months 'Directly Observed Treatment, Short course' taken at home for tuberculosis, while he continues with the AIDS treatment. He has gained weight, is not anaemic anymore, the itchy skin rash has disappeared and his CD4 cell count is at 400 cells per mm^3. And most importantly Ramesh feels well. He is back at work in the corner shop.

Although the financial resources available for tuberculosis and HIV/AIDS control have increased remarkably over the last decade, not enough headway has been made and progress will remain limited unless overall health systems are strengthened, and the vertical focus on tuberculosis or HIV/AIDS is combined with the horizontal strengthening of the health system. The world has the financial and technological resources to bring essential health services to all. The existing methods for combating tuberculosis and HIV/AIDS, although imperfect, are adequate to greatly reduce the effect of these diseases. However, the woeful state of health systems in many poor countries thwarts these effective interventions, including prevention, from reaching those in greatest need, even where resources are available. Until systems are in place to deliver essential health services on a large scale, attempts to address individual diseases will flounder, and progress against one will be bought at the price of neglecting others. Although global political and financial commitment for disease control has grown, far more attention and a greater share of resources must be invested in building and strengthening health systems as a whole.

Sources and suggestions for further reading

For the history of tuberculosis and HIV I made use of Roy Porter's *The Greatest Benefit to Mankind: A Medical History of Humanity* (W.W. Norton & Company, London, 1997), as well as David Weatherall's *Science and the Quiet Art: The Role of Medical Research in Health Care* (W.W. Norton & Company, New York, 1995). Michael and Linda Hutcheon describe in *Opera Desire, Disease, Death* (University of Nebraska Press, 1996), a book about seeing illnesses through opera glasses, the cultural and historical change in the cases of Mimi in *La Bohème* and Violetta in *La Traviata*. Gary Maartens and Robert Wilkinson described the epidemiology, diagnosis, treatment and control of tuberculosis in a review ('seminar') paper in *The Lancet* (2007; 370: 2030–2043), while these different aspects are also discussed in a special theme issue (May 2007) on tuberculosis in the *Bulletin of the World Health Organization*. As an example of a successful country programme, the very impressive results of 10-year experience in DOTS expansion and implementation in China is described in a paper by Xianyi Chen and others (*Bulletin of the World Health Organization* 2002; 80: 430–436). A series of six papers about HIV prevention was published in *The Lancet* in August/September 2008, emphasizing the importance of combination prevention and the importance of biomedical, behavioural and structural strategies. Elizabeth Pisani argues in her book *The Wisdom of Whores: Bureaucrats, Brothels and the Business of AIDS* (Granta, London and Norton, New York, 2008), that a substantial proportion of the funding devoted to HIV/AIDS is wasted on ineffective programming, the result of science and good public health policy being trumped by politics, ideology and morality. The book is flawed in some of its argumentation, but is a great read. For a review of the vast divide between rich and poor countries in the prevention and treatment options for HIV in children, as well as solutions to this problem, see the paper by K. E. Little and others in *Tropical Medicine and International Health* (2008; 13: 1098–1110). In a special issue of the Journal *AIDS and*

Behaviour (July 2006; 10) in an editorial by Michael Merson, as well as several other articles, the multiple factors contributing to the decline in HIV prevalence in Uganda are discussed.

4
Safe motherhood

... how many of us realize that, in much of the world, the act of giving birth to a child is still the biggest killer of women of child-bearing age?

Liya Kebede, 2005

There are stories in many poor countries of women who tell their older children when the delivery is approaching that 'she is going on a long journey from which she may not return ...',

Anonymous, 2003

Pendo

She stares straight in front of her. We have just told Pendo that she is cured and that she can go home. After four weeks in hospital and a major operation, Pendo is not incontinent of urine anymore and she will be able to live the life of a 'normal' woman.

Pendo had been married at the age of fourteen, she became pregnant soon after that, and stayed in the village and hut of her husband's family to deliver her firstborn. Without doubt her mother-in-law encouraged her strongly to push well to get the baby out and to make no noise. When Pendo, after three days of strong contractions hadn't delivered, she was transported to the closest hospital, 50 km away from her village. In the hospital a caesarean section was performed, the baby was born in poor condition and died the same day.

Pendo had a slow and difficult recovery from the operation, had a severe infection, and was incontinent of urine. The prolonged pressure of the head of the baby was the cause of a large hole or fistula between Pendo's bladder and the birth canal. After two years of seeking health care for her problem in many places, Pendo arrived at Sumve hospital in north-west Tanzania, far away from her village and family. She had heard that in our hospital women with her problem could be cured. She was operated upon and became 'dry'. During the period of Pendo's admission she was cared for by the nurses and fellow patients. If you asked Pendo when her family would come to visit her, she always said 'labda kesho' – 'perhaps tomorrow'. Her family never came. Pendo had been rejected by her husband, his family and her own family. Her father had to return the dowry, composed of 20 cows, to her in-laws. Pendo had failed, she had not and would not 'produce' children and she smelled.

Vesicovaginal fistula

Vesicovaginal fistula is a devastating injury in which an abnormal opening forms between a woman's bladder and vagina, resulting in urinary incontinence because the urine passes uncontrollably via the vagina. As with leprosy, and when it becomes clear that the constant loss of urine (or faeces when there is a fistula between the rectum and the vagina) is a chronic condition, these women are often divorced or abandoned by their husbands and relatives. Additionally, as the cause of fistula is not readily apparent to the surrounding community, they may view these injuries as a punishment from God for sexual misbehaviour or as a form of venereal disease, and blame the victim for her predicament and with that add further to her social stigmatization. Frequently these women are also mourning the loss of a baby after prolonged labour. Depression, anxiety and other forms of mental health dysfunction are common among women with vesicovaginal fistula. In rich countries, such fistulas are rare, and arise mainly from malignant disease, radiation therapy or surgical injury – usually to the bladder during hysterectomy. In the poor countries of Africa and south Asia, however, vesicovaginal fistulas are a common problem, afflicting many women. It is estimated that more than 2 million women in poor countries have unrepaired vesicovaginal fistulas, and 50,000–100,000 new cases develop each year. In these countries, fistulas are usually caused by prolonged obstructed labour, which was also once the most common cause of fistulas in Europe and the US. Fistula from obstructed labour was eradicated from rich countries by the middle of the 20th century as effective systems of obstetric care were developed to cover the entire population of childbearing women.

Labour becomes obstructed when a woman cannot deliver her baby through her birth canal because of a discrepancy between the size of the baby's head and the space available in her pelvis. Two major evolutionary forces have made human females very susceptible to this cephalo-pelvic disproportion. The assumption of an upright posture and bipedal gait has imposed structural constraints on the architecture of the human pelvis, and the size of the human brain and hence of the head has increased over time. The problem of cephalo-pelvic disproportion is especially prevalent in parts of the world where girls grow up malnourished, marry early and become pregnant before they have achieved full pelvic growth. The problem faced by women experiencing obstructed labour must be solved by surgery – caesarean section or operative vaginal delivery but timely access to essential obstetric services is often non-existent in poor countries, especially in rural areas.

Virtually all obstetric fistulas could be prevented by adequate delivery care that detects abnormal progression of labour and allow intervention before the labour becomes obstructed. Simple graphic analysis of the progress of labour with the use of the partograph by trained birth attendants prevents prolonged labour, results in a decrease in operative interventions by allowing normal labour to proceed without unnecessary interference, and reduces maternal deaths. Yet, even this level of basic obstetric care is often absent in poor countries. Unfortunately, the provision of delivery care is often not a top priority for the governments of countries where the fistula problem is most severe. Furthermore, the backlog of unrepaired fistulas continues to increase in these countries.

The basic techniques needed for fistula repair have been known since the 1840s, when James Marion Sims accomplished his first successful corrections in Alabama, US, on slave-women. More recent advances in fistula surgery have come in the areas of improved anaesthesia, synthetic suture materials, better urinary catheters, earlier repair and techniques of tissue grafting, rather than from breakthroughs in basic science. Fistulas can be repaired at minimum cost with relatively low-technology surgical operations done under spinal surgery, and can be performed even by trained non-doctors with good manual dexterity. However, the possession of surgical skills is not enough. Many other problems are associated with providing fistula repair services in poor countries. As was the case with Pendo, fistula sufferers tend to be young, illiterate, destitute women from rural areas, without political influence or economic resources. Very often these women cannot pay even the modest rates charged at hospitals in poor countries. And the necessity for prolonged catheter drainage after surgery (10–14 days) to permit the bladder to heal means that fistula patients require longer hospital stays and more intensive nursing than many other surgical patients – which can make them unpopular with nursing staff. Furthermore, fistula cases are rarely emergencies. In hospitals that provide general surgical services, scheduled fistula cases are frequently bumped from the operating lists because of road traffic accidents or other emergencies. It is estimated that since 2003 less than 12,000 women have received fistula surgery in Asia and Africa. As with leper colonies and because of the stigma of the disease, fistula surgery seems to be most efficiently done in specialized centres dedicated exclusively to the care of women with vesicovaginal fistulas. Good examples of such centres exist in Ethiopia and Nigeria. One additional advantage of specialized fistula hospitals where large numbers of women can be treated, is that they allow for the development of a unique care model where much of the nursing, including psychosocial care and support is provided by current or former fistula patients.

In general, fistula patients are not high priority in health care systems of poor countries. They are at the bottom of the heap socially, sexually, economically, politically and medically. And one can probably say the same for safe motherhood – the international aid community has been largely uninterested in funding programmes that provide essential obstetric services for the poor women in the world. In 2002 it was estimated that maternal health services represented just 5–11 per cent of total donor contributions to the health sector in poor countries, and 4–12 per cent of domestic health expenditure. As a result, many have come to regard 'safe motherhood' as an 'orphan initiative'.

Measuring maternal mortality

The maternal mortality data in many poor countries are inadequate and the women who lose their lives as a result of pregnancy and childbirth essentially remain invisible to the governments and agencies who determine policy. For this to be seen as a priority requires strong advocates armed with strong data.

Wendy Graham, 2002

Today a woman's risk of dying of pregnancy-related causes in the poorest countries is still estimated to be higher than it was more than a century ago in the richest nations. A 100-fold disparity exists between maternal mortality ratios in rich countries and those in the poorest countries; 99 per cent of the world's estimated 536,000 maternal deaths per year occur in the so-called developing world – and there is no public health indicator where the disparity between rich and poor countries is as large as for maternal mortality. As shown in Figure 4.1, and in comparison with Figure 2.3, countries with high levels of

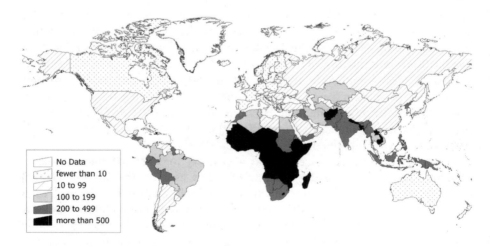

Figure 4.1 *Map showing the global distribution of maternal mortality ratios (per 100,000 live births)*

Source: Millenium Development Goals Indicators. The official United Nations site for the MDG indicators at mdgs.un.org/unsd/mdg (accessed on 16 February 2010)

maternal mortality predominate in the same regions where countries are poor. The disparity is even greater when a woman's life-time risk of dying as the result of a complication of pregnancy or childbirth is considered. For example, a woman's lifetime risk of dying as the result of a pregnancy-related cause is estimated to be 1 in 29,800 in Sweden, but as high as 1 in 7 or 8 for Afghanistan, Niger and Sierra Leone. This is despite high levels of awareness among governments and international agencies that the vast majority of maternal deaths are avoidable. It is also in spite of the Safe Motherhood Initiative that was launched more than 20 years ago. As Wendy Graham, Professor of Obstetric Epidemiology at the University of Aberdeen, has argued, for this to be seen as a priority requires strong advocates armed with strong data.The data we have for levels and trends in maternal mortality for many poor countries are inadequate, and the effectiveness and cost-effectiveness of intervention strategies are not well worked out. Action needs to be informed by an understanding of who is dying, when, where and why.

History of maternal mortality in Sweden, England and Wales, and the US

> *No variation in the health of the states of Europe is the result of chance; it is the direct result of physical and political conditions in which nations live.*
>
> William Farr, 1866

Around 1870, maternal mortality ratios in what are now rich countries were above 600 per 100,000 live births. For some of these countries – such as Sweden, England and Wales, and the US – detailed time series are available. These show different patterns of reduction. Swedish maternal mortality ratios started dropping as early as the 1870s and stabilized at 250–300 per 100,000 live births around the turn of the century; at that time England and Wales were still at levels of 400–450 and the US at 600–800, and they remained unchanged for another four decades (see Figure 4.2). This period of stagnation was followed by fast reduction, between the mid-1930s and 1960, which brought all these countries to around 20–30 per 100,000 live births. How can the differences be explained?

From 1749 onwards Sweden had a General Register for the systematic collection of individual health data, and as early as 1751 the Swedish Health Commission directed attention towards 'avoidable maternal mortality' with the observation that at least 400 women of 651 dying during childbirth could have been saved if only there had been enough trained midwives. The health authorities consequently developed a policy of training enough professional midwives to ensure that qualified personnel would attend all births, which mainly took place at home. In 1861 professional midwives attended 40 per cent of births, and by 1900 the proportion had risen to 78 per cent – while only 2–5 per cent of births took place at the hospital. The organizational

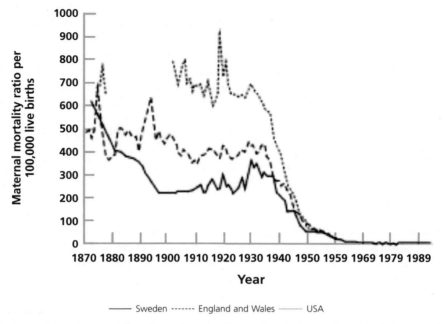

Figure 4.2 *Evolution of maternal mortality in Sweden, England & Wales and the USA from 1870–1993*

Source: de Brouwere, V. et al. *Tropical Medicine & International Health* 1998: 3; 771–782

development went along with the prompt introduction of modern techniques; certified midwives were allowed to use forceps as early as 1829. But the major decline in maternal mortality occurred after the implementation of aseptic techniques. These had been introduced in hospitals in the late 1870s, and by 1881 all certified midwives had been instructed to apply this new technology. The early adoption of the combination of professional assistance to home deliveries and the use of effective techniques supported by political commitment enabled Sweden to achieve its relatively low maternal mortality ratios by the beginning of the 20th century.

Between 1850 and 1930 in England and Wales, maternal mortality ratios remained well above what Sweden had achieved by that time. Awareness of the problem came much later than in Sweden. It was only in 1928 that a special committee appointed by the Ministry of Health put forward the concept of a 'primary avoidable factor' among the causes of maternal mortality, 77 years later than in Sweden. By 1935, maternal mortality ratios began to fall, mainly as a result of a steady decline in puerperal infections. During the 1940s the capacity to handle major emergencies in a hospital environment further decreased levels, down to 85 in 1950. It was not until 1949 however that confidential enquiries into maternal deaths drew attention to other causes of maternal mortality that could be avoided by effective methods of prevention and treatment. With the development of this new knowledge, and under strong pressure from the public, both obstetric specialists and primary care givers became aware of their potential to reduce maternal mortality and managed to assess needs for improvements, for example, control of bleeding, safe anaesthesia and effective emergency obstetric services. These enquiries played the part of a medical audit, and the resulting awareness among caregivers largely contributed to the decline: from 85 to 25 per 100,000 live births between 1950 and 1965.

In the US reliable vital statistics became available in the 1920s, much later than in Sweden or England. The available data show that in 1918 maternal mortality in the US was 885 per 100,000 live births, as high as Sweden a century before and twice the Swedish ratio before the mid-19th century. Increasing public interest in the problem of maternal mortality and reports such as the one published in 1933 by the New York Academy of Medicine resulted in actions that led to a declining trend from the late 1930s onwards. These actions included investments in professional midwifery training and referral hospitals, asepsis for the prevention of puerperal infections, a supportive system with regulation and legislation, control and supervision of the medical and midwifery profession, and information to confirm progress.

From this we can learn that a large reduction in the maternal mortality ratio is achievable within a relatively short timeframe. The enormous difference between Sweden with a maternal mortality ratio of 300 per 100,000 live births in 1935 and the US with 600 deaths per 100,000 live births was essentially eliminated by 1960, when many rich countries reached ratios of 20–30 deaths per 100,000 live births. Thus, to reduce by three-quarters the maternal mortality ratio within a 25-year timeframe – one of the targets of Millennium Development Goal 5 – is achievable. Evidence from poorer countries including Bangladesh, Egypt, Honduras, Malaysia, Sri Lanka and Thailand over the last few decades also suggests that a 75 per cent decline is feasible.

When, where and why do women die?

Most maternal deaths seem to occur between the third trimester of pregnancy and the first week after delivery. Mortality can be extremely high especially in the first two days after birth. The direct consequences of pregnancy and childbirth continue to account for most maternal deaths in poor countries. Haemorrhage, hypertensive diseases and infections are often the most common causes, followed by obstructed labour and abortion. Although this pattern is common, underrepresentation is likely due to a lack of good quality data and the difficulty of gathering information on some causes – for example, complications from illegally induced abortions.

Haemorrhage is a major cause of maternal mortality in poor countries, and arguably the most preventable. Attempts to reduce deaths from haemorrhage have been complicated by the fact that many deaths occur in out-of-hospital settings, that death may occur within a short period of time before transfer to a health facility is possible, and that primary methods of prevention and treatment depend on access to timely and competent obstetric care that needs to be available 24 hours a day and seven days a week. The proportion of deaths attributable to induced and unsafe abortions is not known, and is likely to be underestimated especially in countries where abortion is illegal or restricted.

The contribution to maternal deaths of diseases that are not unique to pregnancy – the so-called indirect causes – is also largely unknown in poor countries, partly due to poor diagnostic capability and partly because pregnancies are often not reported for such causes. An increased susceptibility to a number of infections occurs during pregnancy, probably as a consequence of down-regulation of the immune system in an attempt to protect the foetus. AIDS especially, and also malaria and tuberculosis, seem to be important indirect, and underestimated causes of maternal mortality in many poor countries. In the countries most severely affected by HIV, such as Malawi, Zimbabwe and South Africa, the HIV epidemic is thought to have reversed previous gains in maternal mortality reduction.

The clustering of maternal mortality around delivery, and the importance of haemorrhage, hypertensive disorders, infections and obstructed labour as causes of death, means that all women should have access to skilled birth attendance at birth and immediately after that, and timely referral for emergency care. Where maternal mortality is highest, there are severe access problems to such care, a scarcity of skilled staff and often relatively excessive costs for mothers – and therefore substantial barriers to progress.

Poor–rich inequities in professional delivery care are much larger than other forms of care such as professional antenatal care, childhood immunization and medical treatment for childhood illnesses. There are not only differences between countries, but also very important differences within countries – delivery care by professional birth attendants favours the relatively rich in most poor countries. Poor–rich inequalities are also large within both rural and urban areas, but for the most part births without professional delivery care occur among the rural poor. A similar pattern can be seen for life-saving caesarean sections. It is assumed that in any population at least 1 per cent of all pregnant women need a surgical delivery to save their lives, and in the poorest countries large segments of the population have caesarean section rates below 1 per cent. Within countries there are again large poor–rich inequalities for this indicator, and the situation is worse in the rural compared to the urban areas.

For both delivery care by professional birth attendants and life-saving caesarean sections this disparity is related to demand and supply factors of maternity care. There are often strong beliefs and practices around pregnancy and childbirth in local communities and societies, and cultural factors may be more important determinants of the demand for maternity care than other types of care. Poorer women often prefer traditional birth attendants or family members, especially if childbirth is seen as a non-illness event where modern medicine has little to contribute. Professional providers of maternity care may not be tolerant of cultural beliefs and practices. It is too often the case that professional providers treat poor women with less consideration than wealthier or more educated women. Also, women can experience constraints in seeking professional health care if relatives, especially husbands and mothers-in-law, are heavily involved in or determine the decision-making process. Families might be less willing to spend money on women's health in some societies, while male doctors may be an important barrier to seeking facility-based delivery care. In contrast, richer, often better educated, women and their families more frequently have a more modern world view, greater identification with modern health systems, increased confidence in dealing with health professionals and officials, and a greater ability and willingness to travel outside their community, all of which facilitate the use of professional maternity care and delivery at a health facility.

On the supply side, lack of availability and accessibility is greater for professional delivery care than for many other forms of care. The physical infrastructure requirements are higher for facility-based delivery than for the provision of vaccinations or the medical treatment of common childhood illnesses. Moreover, providers of vaccinations and the treatment of common childhood illnesses can include lower-level cadres, such as community health workers, who are more easily placed in remote and rural areas than doctors or midwives. Finally, more immunizations or treatment of common child illnesses can be done per provider per day than deliveries. The human resources crisis in the health sector of poor countries is particularly affecting professional delivery care services. There are an estimated 60 million deliveries per year unassisted by professional health workers. Assuming that a single midwife can assist 150 births annually – while also providing antenatal and often neglected postnatal care – this means that an additional 400,000 midwives need to be trained and posted. These professional midwives will require salaries, housing and allowances for posting in rural areas, work opportunities for their spouses, and educational facilities for their children. There is also a need for continuing education and supervision, and the possibility to refer and transport patients for timely access to advanced emergency obstetric care.

A lack of affordability might explain in part the large poor–rich inequalities in both professional delivery attendance and life-saving caesarean sections within urban and rural areas. On the other hand there is also the increasing problem of 'overuse' of caesarean sections, including 'on request' interventions, especially in urban settings, exposing mothers and babies to unnecessary harm and expense and taking away sparse resources from where they are really needed. The cost of delivery care can be an important barrier. The time spent looking for cash can also delay access to emergency life-saving care in facilities. Even where this service is officially free, hidden costs such as transport costs and lost time by women and relatives in order to receive health care may add up to a substantial part of monthly income, or even several times one family's monthly income. Moreover, the costs of facility-based delivery can be unpredictable and the treatment of severe complications can have a catastrophic impact on household budgets (up to the annual income or more for poor families). Poor–rich inequalities may also increase when services require action at a very specific point in time. Delivery care has a short time window in which effective care can be sought, in contrast to, for instance, antenatal care and immunization, for which more time is available.

A call for action

Where is the M in MCH (Maternal and Child Health)?
Allan Rosenfield and Deborah Maine, 1985

The large inequalities in maternity care underline the need for effective and user-friendly provision of affordable services, which is mainly about overcoming health system constraints. Governments and the international community must recognize that the reduction of maternal mortality is a long-term effort with no single solution or 'magic bullet'. With complex challenges working through health systems, any acceleration in progress will require long-term support. A team of the Health Economics and Financing Programme of the London School of Hygiene and Tropical Medicine recently reported that donor disbursements for maternal and neonatal health – (increasingly the two are combined as the association of the presence of a skilled attendant and timely access to emergency care with neonatal deaths is similar to those for maternal deaths) – increased from US$704 million in 2003 to almost $1.2 billion in 2006, representing just 1 per cent of gross development assistance disbursements. This translates into an increase from $7 per birth in 2003 to $12 per birth in 2006. Unfortunately, the analysis also showed that, in contrast to child health where countries with higher child mortality receive more development aid (overall allocation was $2.3 billion in 2006 for child health), assistance to maternal and neonatal health (in 2008 more than 40 per cent of all children who died before their fifth birthday died in the first month, and half of these before they were a few days old) does not seem to be well targeted towards countries with the greatest maternal health needs. And, although expenditures are increasing, it is far from sufficient – an increase to an estimated $6.1 billion is needed to increase coverage to desired levels to achieve safe motherhood for all.

In September 2000, 189 countries pledged to support the Millennium Development Goals, including the target to reduce by three-quarters maternal mortality ratios. Safe motherhood is an important poverty eradication strategy, as improved maternal health services, which are available equitably, can help not only to reduce the gap in the numbers of maternal deaths between rich and poor people, but also reduce the economic impact on poor families, both of catastrophic payments owing to emergency care and of the death or disability of (often) the most important member of the household. Governments can and should adopt policies to protect the poorest families from the catastrophic consequences of unaffordable delivery charges. In addition, if they haven't done so already, governments should plan for the training and deployment of the required human resources, especially midwives, as well as in efforts to retain existing staff. This should include discouragement of the international brain drain by improving working conditions and offering appropriate incentives for good quality maternity care.

Rapid progress to reduce maternal mortality, 'near-miss events' (severe pregnancy or childbirth-related complications that nearly cause death), and long-term disabilities is possible, but much more can and must be done. Improved maternal health care, especially around the delivery and immediately after giving birth, can make a difference – but there is also a need to improve the education of women and men, improve the livelihoods and the status of women, and strengthen civil society within an overall development agenda. These actions are medium- to long-term, but they can provide enabling conditions for more proximate interventions (such as the creation of demand for skilled delivery care) that will help to increase the effect of, and sustain, the health systems interventions. Pendo was young, illiterate, destitute, without political influence or economic resources, and in the absence of these factors it would have been very unlikely that she would have suffered a vesicovaginal fistula and experienced the death of her child. Delivery care cannot remain a Cinderella service for poor women in many parts of the world. It is the joint and individual responsibility of health care workers, researchers, advocates and policy- and decision-makers, to act.

Sources and suggestions for further reading

Lewis Wall's review paper: 'Obstetric vesicovaginal fistula as an international public health problem', published in *The Lancet* (2006; 368: 1201–1209) , is an excellent introduction to the vesicovaginal fistula problem. For the treatment of vesicovaginal fistulas I consulted J. B. Lawson and D. B. Stewart's *Obstetrics and Gynaecology in the Tropics and Developing Countries*, first published by Edward Arnold in 1967 which remained in print until 1991 and now, unfortunately, has become a collectors' item. A fact sheet on obstetric fistula is available at www.who.int/features/factfiles/obstetric_fistula/en/index.html (accessed 11 March 2010). For the history of the reduction of maternal mortality in Sweden, England and Wales, and the US, I made good use of the detailed analyses by Vincent de Brouwere et al. 'Strategies for reducing maternal mortality in developing countries: What can we learn from the history of the industrialized West?' in *Tropical Medicine & International Health* (1998; 3: 771–782), and Irvine Loudon's *Death in Childbirth* (Oxford: Clarendon Press, 1992). The 2006 *Lancet* Maternal Health Series, especially the papers by Carine Ronsmans et al. 'Maternal mortality: Who, when, where and why', (2006; 368: 1189–1200), and Veronique Filippi et al. 'Maternal health in poor countries: The broader context and a call for action', (2006;

368: 1535–1541), give a detailed account of the current state of the subject. On the poor–rich differences in maternal mortality I have also drawn heavily on the paper by Tanja Houweling et al. 'Huge poor–rich inequalities in maternity care: An international comparative study of maternity and child care in developing countries', in *Bulletin of the World Health Organization* (2007; 85: 745–754). The figures quoted in the text of donor disbursements for maternal and neonatal health can be found back in Giulia Greco and others, 'Countdown to 2015: Assessment of donor assistance to maternal, newborn, and child health between 2003 and 2006', *The Lancet* (2008; 371: 1268–1275), while Wendy Graham's call for better maternal mortality data is in 'Now or never: The case for measuring maternal mortality', *The Lancet* (2002; 359: 701–704). New analysis published online on 12 April 2010 by Margaret Hogan and others in *The Lancet* indicated that the global number of maternal deaths had fallen from 526,300 in 1980 to 342,900 in 2008 (and corrected the 2005 estimate of 535,900). Although there are wide uncertainty intervals around these numbers, which were expected to provoke intense debate among maternal mortality measurement experts, the overall message is one of welcome progress. *Investing in Maternal Health: Learning from Malaysia and Sri Lanka* by Indra Pathmanathan and colleagues, as well as *Reducing Maternal Mortality: Learning from Bolivia, China, Egypt, Honduras, Indonesia, Jamaica and Zimbabwe* edited by Marjorie Koblinski, contain success stories and lessons learned from low- and middle-income countries (Washington DC: both published by the World Bank in 2003).

5
Family planning

Those who in principle oppose birth control are either incapable of arithmetic or else in favour of war, pestilence and famine as permanent features of human life.

Bertrand Russell, 1928

Kaddy

Kaddy, a 30-year-old remarried divorcee, living in the Farafenni area in The Gambia, had a sad reproductive history. Kaddy had had four pregnancies. Three were with her first husband. The first pregnancy resulted in a daughter who died before the age of three, and pregnancies number two and three both resulted in stillbirths. At this point Kaddy's marriage ended, very likely as a consequence of her failure to produce heirs for her first husband. Kaddy remarried as the marginal second wife of a man already married to a younger woman with three children. Kaddy became pregnant for a fourth time and bore a son for her new husband. Kaddy was interviewed for the first time as a participant in a 1992–1995 research project on family planning and birth intervals in rural Gambia, when her baby was about 17 months old. Four months later, this child died. Left in an insecure marriage with no children to support her in later life, Kaddy, still expressing a resolute desire for more children, did the last thing one might expect. She started on injectable contraception.

Kaddy's case was not unusual, in the study 18 per cent of women who were using modern contraceptives, did so after a reproductive health 'mishap', meaning that their last pregnancy ended in a miscarriage, a stillbirth or the death of a young child. This finding might seem surprising in a rural uneducated West African community whose members place high value on fertility (on average, women in this community had seven births over the course of their lifetimes). It is not. Traditional cultures have long understood that births need to be sufficiently spaced for a woman's health and 'vitality' to be preserved and replenished. That is why there are so many cultural practices that different communities use to modulate human conception. In some of these settings, birth control methods are used much less to reduce the number of children than to space them.

The history of birth control

When the history of civilization is written, it will be a biological history and Margaret Sanger will be its heroine

H.G. Wells, 1935

Probably the oldest methods of contraception (aside from sexual abstinence and extended breastfeeding) were *coitus interruptus*, certain barrier methods and herbal methods. *Coitus interruptus*, withdrawal of the penis from the vagina prior to ejaculation, probably predates any other form of birth control. Once the relationship between the emission of semen into the vagina and pregnancy was suspected, some men began using this technique. There are historic records of Egyptian women using a pessary made of various acidic substances and lubricated with honey or oil, which might have been somewhat effective in killing sperm. During the medieval period, physicians in the Islamic world listed many birth control substances in their medical encyclopaedias. The condom appeared sometime in the 17th century, and was initially made of animal intestine. It was not particularly popular, nor as effective as modern latex condoms, but was employed both as a means of contraception and in the hope of avoiding syphilis, which was greatly feared and devastating prior to the discovery of antibiotics.

The fact that various methods of birth control were known in the ancient world sharply contrasts with a seeming ignorance of these methods in wide segments of the population of early modern Christian Europe. This ignorance continued far into the 20th century, and was accompanied with high birth rates in Europe during the 18th and 19th centuries. Between 1750 and 1850 Britain's population increased threefold, from around 6 million to 18 million. London had about 800,000 inhabitants in 1801, by 1841 its population had grown by a further one million, and at the death of Queen Victoria in 1901 it contained seven million inhabitants. The London story was repeated with a time lag throughout the evolving industrialized world.

Thomas Malthus, an English cleric and pioneering political economist, made his famously grim prediction in an essay on population, first published in 1798, that gains in food production could not keep up with natural population increase. Malthus' views have subsequently been variously contested or supported by other economists. Some economists writing mainly in the 1980s, with Julian Simon of the US as most prominent proponent, promoted the idea that humans are themselves a 'resource' – the more humans, the more likely it is that invention and innovation will flow. In contrast, economists familiar with ecological realities recognize that there are fundamental limits to the Earth's capacity in that it is essentially a closed system within which the continuing and sustainable increases in food production cannot be assumed. As a man of his time and setting, Malthus advocated delayed marriage and strict premarital chastity, which he called moral restraint, for birth control. The strict European approach to contraception was later carried to the 'New World'. The anti-contraceptive bias, with a base in protection of family morals as well as a puritanical attitude remained mainstream for a long time. In 1877, on the eve of England's fertility decline, Charles Bradlaugh and Annie Besant were brought to trial in London for distributing a pamphlet on birth control. In 1916, Margaret Sanger was arrested for opening a birth control clinic in Brooklyn, New York. Sanger worked as a nurse in the tenements of New York, and was deeply disturbed by the misery and suffering she found in large immigrant families. Having observed the death of a woman due to criminal abortion she resolved 'to do something to change the destiny of mothers' and espoused the birth control cause. Her many arrests and prosecutions, and the resulting outcries, helped lead to changes in laws allowing doctors to give birth control advice (and later, birth control devices) to patients.

The first modern intrauterine device ('IUD') was described in a German publication in 1908. The Gräfenberg ring, the first IUD to be used by a significant number of women, was introduced in 1928. The rhythm method was developed in the early 20th century, as researchers discovered that a woman only ovulates once per menstrual cycle. Not until the 1950s, when scientists better understood the functioning of the menstrual cycle and the hormones that controlled it, were methods of hormonal contraception and modern methods of fertility awareness (also called 'natural family planning') developed. In 1959 the US Food and Drug Administration approved the first form of hormonal birth control, the combined oral contraceptive pill. 'The pill', comprising progestin and oestrogen, essentially acts by mimicking the body's own production of sex hormones. The amount of oestrogen contained in the pill was not well studied in safety trials, and in the 1960s women were seriously overdosed. By 1969, adverse side-effects including thrombosis, phlebitis, migraine and jaundice were being reported, and in 1969 the UK Committee on the Safety of Medicines advised the prescription of oral contraceptives with no more than 50 microgrammes of oestrogen. The safe low-dose pill or the progestins only pill (also known as the 'mini-pill') are now the standard.

Programmes to promote family planning in poor countries started in the 1960s in response to improvements in child survival, which in turn led to rapid population growth. In Asian countries, the main motive was often to enhance the prospects of socio-economic growth by reducing population growth, and governments took the lead. In Latin America, initiatives were mostly started as a response to increases in criminal abortions, and efforts to remedy the situation by providing access to modern contraceptives were led by nongovernmental organizations. The number of low- and middle-income countries with official policies to support family planning rose from only two in 1960 to 115 by 1996. International funding increased in parallel from US$168 million in 1971 to $560 million in 1995. Success in boosting contraceptive use and reducing fertility was slow to come but, by 1990, reproductive change was established throughout most of Latin America and Asia, including some of the world's poorest countries at that time such as Bangladesh and Nepal, and fertility decline had begun in most sub-Saharan African regions.

Success came at a price. Family planning strategies in some Asian countries such as the ones in China, India and Vietnam were criticized as coercive and the quality of services in many low- and middle-income countries were deemed unsatisfactory. These concerns came to the fore at the fifth International Population Conference held in Cairo in 1994. The recommendations of the Cairo conference replaced the dominant demographic-economic rationale for family planning programmes with a broader agenda encompassing women's empowerment and reproductive health and rights. Despite the enthusiasm generated by the Cairo conference, family planning has dropped steadily down the list of international development priorities since 1994. By 2003, donor support for family planning commodities and service delivery had reduced to $460 million. Those who drafted the Millennium Development Goals in 2000 ignored the difficulties posed by sustained rapid population growth in many of the world's poorest countries and thus family planning was not included as a goal. Population growth and family planning are now often marginalized in key reports.

Population growth, demographic transition, and carrying capacity

Between 1960 and 2005, the global population rose by 114 per cent, from 3 billion to nearly 6.5 billion. In Figure 5.1 the total fertility (children per woman) per country is shown; countries with high fertility predominate where countries are poor. Over the next 45 years, the percentage increase is expected to be much lower (40 per cent) but will still remain very large in absolute numbers (2.6 billion). These figures assume that fertility in Asia and Latin America will fall from 2.4 to slightly below 2.0 births per woman and that in sub-Saharan Africa fertility will drop steadily from 5.0 births to about 2.5 births by 2050. Under these assumptions, the world population is expected to be a little over 9 billion in 2050. Half the expected increase will come from Asia and 36 per cent from sub-Saharan Africa. However, if fertility is half a birth higher or lower over the 45 years between 2005 and 2050, the global population will reach 10.6 or 7.7 billion, respectively, by 2050. Three factors account for future population growth. The first one relates to the fact that the birth rate is sustained at a raised level because of the high proportion of the population in the reproductive age range. The effect of this will gradually diminish as populations age, but between now and 2050 the young populations in many poor countries will account for more than half of the projected increase in the world's population. The second factor is unwanted births (a result of unmet need for contraception). Elimination of such births could reduce population growth by about 20 per cent. The third factor is high desired family size; many couples report that they want more children than the number that will eventually allow the population size to stabilize. This factor also accounts for about 20 per cent of population growth, but more in Africa where desired family sizes are still very high.

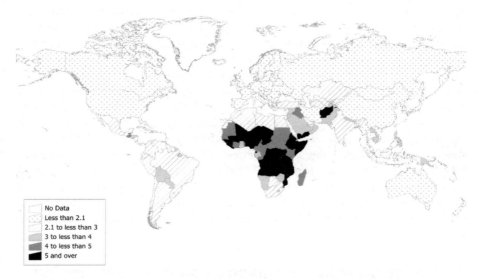

No Data
Less than 2.1
2.1 to less than 3
3 to less than 4
4 to less than 5
5 and over

Figure 5.1 *Map showing the global distribution of total fertility (children per woman)*

Source: United Nations Department of Economic and Social Affairs, Population Division, United Nations World Population Prospects: 2006 Revision. New York, U.N., 2007

The term demographic transition was first used in 1945 to describe the changes in birth and death rates that have historically accompanied the shift from a traditional to a 'modern' society. With modernization, indicating social and economic development, sharp declines in mortality have been followed by a reduction in fertility, although usually lagging by years or decades. The term transition refers to a shift away from a stable, high-stationary stage of population in which very high birth rates are balanced by very high death rates and there is no or little population growth. As a society undergoes modernization, there is a transition with falling mortality, especially in child mortality, but with continued high birth rates leading to explosive population growth. Birth rates then tend to drop, and a new, low-stationary state is reached in which birth and death rates are low and balance resumes. The end result is a striking change in the age structure of the population, with fewer children and an ageing population. These population changes are reflected in the shift from a wide-based pyramid, with large numbers in the younger age groups, to a structure with a narrow base, nearly rectangular in configuration, and nearly equal percentages in each age group (see Figure 5.2).

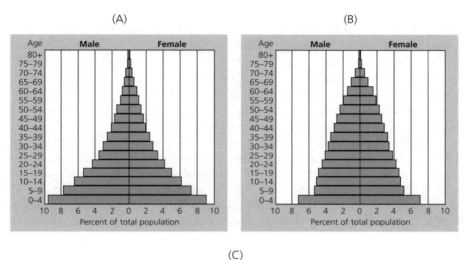

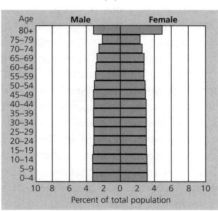

Figure 5.2 *The demographic transition*

(A) high fertility/high mortality; (B) high fertility/declining mortality; (C) low fertility/low mortality.

Source: Reprinted from U.S. Census Bureau. *International Population Reports WP/02. Global Population Profile: 2007.* Washington D.C., Government Printing Office, 2004: 35

Historically, all countries that have undergone modernization with a marked drop in child mortality have had rapid population growth. In the past, this population growth has always been followed by falling fertility rates, but its form and timescale have so far been situation-dependent. In some countries, such as The Netherlands, birth rates remained high long after death rates fell.

Industrializing Europe in the late 18th and 19th centuries was able to alleviate the pressures of its expanding populations via large emigrations to North America and less so, to Australia and New Zealand. In China, a gradual slow decline in death rates began as early as the 17th century. This has been variously attributed to the production of higher-yielding crops, improved agricultural practices, immunization against smallpox and the introduction of basic family and community hygiene. Elsewhere in the world the demographic transition has generally begun more recently and has followed a range of paths. Over the past half century many poor countries were able to reduce their infant and child mortality with simple public health and medical interventions. But, on the other hand, fertility decline in several of these countries has been impeded by economic isolation, social conservatism and the retreat of international support for family planning, especially over the last 15 years.

The Population Bomb was a best-selling book written by Paul Ehrlich in 1968. Ehrlich warned of a mass starvation of humans in the 1970s and 1980s due to overpopulation and advocated for immediate action to limit population growth. Maurice King, who in 1966 authored the book *Medical Care in Developing Countries* with groundbreaking work on comprehensive primary health care and health systems in poor countries 'avant la lettre', wrote a controversial paper in 1990 in *The Lancet* on what he termed 'demographic entrapment'. King pointed to a potential major problem that may arise in settings and countries were fertility not to drop. He argued that there is no guarantee that there will be a drop in birth rate in all countries undergoing modernization, and that changes in fertility depend very much on social and cultural characteristics. Demographic entrapment in line with the classic Malthusian scenario would occur in situations in which local, economically isolated and disconnected populations, beset by excessive numbers, cannot feed themselves. Resolution can only be achieved by fratricide, starvation, out-migration or food aid. Some have since argued that complex local crises related to demographic entrapment have occurred in Rwanda and Somalia in the 1990s, and may yet occur in countries such as Burundi, Malawi and parts of South Asia where populations are increasing, land pressures are mounting and environmental conditions including the availability of water are declining. Malthus' original argument was in fact about exceeding 'carrying capacity': situations where there are more people than there is food to feed them. However, unlike other species, human societies typically intervene substantially in the environment in order to increase its carrying capacity. In addition, the hope is that in a better informed and connected world, international cooperation and aid should be able to avert or ameliorate demographic entrapment situations.

Why does family planning still matter?

It is easy to comprehend the idea that rapid growth in a population (often defined as an annual increase of 2 per cent or more, equivalent to a doubling of the population every 34 years) will exacerbate poverty, especially in countries where underemployment is already high and where food security is a concern. In stagnant economies population growth increases the number of poor people – as has happened in sub-Saharan Africa where the estimated number of individuals living on less than a dollar a day rose from 164 million in 1981 to 316 million in 2001. There is good evidence on the benefit of reductions in fertility and population growth. A study of 45 low- and middle-income countries estimated that the proportion of people living in poverty would have fallen by a third if the crude birth rate (number of births per 1000 total population) had decreased by 5 per 1000 population in the 1980s. Fertility decline also brings a long-term benefit. Some 20 years after the onset of the drop in fertility, the proportion of population aged 15–64 starts to rise faster than that of the individuals in less economically productive age ranges. The labour force temporarily grows more rapidly than the population dependent on it, freeing up resources for investment in economic development and family welfare. Other things being equal, per capita income grows more rapidly leading to what has been called the first 'demographic dividend'. This era is then followed a few decades later by a rapid growth in the elderly population. Now, other things being equal, per capita income grows more slowly and the first dividend turns negative. This is the current situation in rich countries – it is the inevitable outcome of high life expectancy and low fertility – but it remains only a distant prospect for poor countries, especially in the rural areas. In addition, a second demographic dividend is also possible. A population concentrated among older working people facing an extended period of retirement has a powerful incentive to accumulate and invest in their assets. The investments transforming into greater assets and sustainable development are not automatic, and as economists argue will depend on the implementation of effective policies.

Within countries there are also large variations in fertility. In 56 low- and middle-income countries, the poorest fifth of women had on average a fertility rate of 6.0 births compared with 3.2 births in the wealthiest fifth. Households with many children are more likely over time to become poor and less likely to recover from poverty than families with few children. Furthermore, children from large families are usually less well nourished and less well educated than those from smaller families. By reaching poor populations with information and services, effective family planning programmes reduce the gap between rich and poor people and can make an important contribution to poverty reduction.

The benefits of family planning for the survival and health of mothers and children are clear. About 90 per cent of global abortion-related and 20 per cent of obstetric-related mortality and morbidity can be averted by the use of effective contraception by women wishing to postpone or cease further childbearing. A total of 150,000 maternal deaths per year can be prevented with high cost-effectiveness and with the largest benefit in the poorest countries. Family planning also brings large health benefits for children, mostly as a result of wider intervals between births. Findings of studies show that conceptions taking place within 18 months of a previous live birth are at the greatest risk of foetal death, low birthweight, prematurity and being small size for gestational age. Evidence suggests that almost one million of the 9.2 million deaths per year of children younger than five years could be averted by combating short birth intervals of less than two years. Effective use of postpartum (and post-abortion) family planning is the most obvious way in which progress towards this ideal could be achieved. Family planning is one of the most cost-effective ways to reduce child mortality and this contribution has been largely overlooked.

Freeing women from involuntary reproduction was one of the main inspirations for family planning pioneers a century ago and remains just as relevant today. The reproductive revolution – the shift from seven births, of whom several might die, to around two births, nearly all of whom survive – represents the most important step towards achieving gender equality by boosting women's opportunities for non-domestic activities. Apart from these socio-economic considerations, contraception allows women to attain the fundamental human right to choose the number and timing of children. Women and men are indispensable partners in family planning, and all people – men and women alike – benefit from information and services. Both men and women need the skills, knowledge and mindset – along with appropriate health care services and supplies – to prevent unintended pregnancies and achieve healthy, intended births. The role of men in family planning is an area that does not get sufficient attention.

The achievement of universal primary education for both sexes is a Millennium Development Goal and many countries also seek to increase secondary-level and tertiary-level enrolments. High fertility and rapid population growth makes this difficult to achieve. Even to maintain existing standards, governments of rapidly growing populations have to double the number of teachers, equipment and classrooms every 20–25 years, and a similar strain is placed on health services. In many countries this has resulted in a drop in expenditure per pupil and a reduction in the quality of education. Universal primary education achieved only at the cost of a decline in the quality of education would be a hollow victory.

Rich nations with low population growth are mainly accountable for the unsustainable exploitation of the world's resources and for threats to the global environment. Poor countries with high rates of population growth have contributed rather little to the carbon dioxide and other emissions that are responsible for global warming. Nevertheless, population growth also threatens the environment. Past growth has had a direct effect on increasing the fraction of land area devoted to food production, with inevitable loss of natural habitats and biodiversity. There is a danger that further population growth in several poor countries will put fragile marginal land under pressure from overcropping and overgrazing, with potentially severe outcomes in terms of loss of vegetation cover, soil fertility depletion and soil erosion. Increasing demand for water is also directly related to population growth, because extra water is needed to grow more food. About one-third of the world's population live under conditions of moderate or severe water stress, a categorization implying that water availability is already, or becoming, a limiting factor. This proportion is bound to rise and could reach two-thirds by 2025. Poor countries will hopefully become richer countries, but with that comes the risk that they will then substantially contribute to degradation of the environment. Increases in CO_2 emissions are very large in the rapidly growing economies of China and India although a significant proportion of their emissions result from the manufacture of goods for rich nations. In a world of 10.6 billion inhabitants, more severe measures are needed to stabilize the planet's environment than for a world of 7.7 billion people. The prevention of unwanted births today via family planning might be one of the most cost-effective ways to preserve the global environment for the future.

What can be done?

Sceptics have argued that 'development is the best contraceptive' and that enhanced living standards and increased life expectancy, education and women's empowerment are the most effective ways to reduce fertility and curb population growth as it will increase demand, although, of course, the supply side is important as well – contraceptive methods should be made available. Family planning proponents argue that reproductive change can be hastened and people's family planning needs met more quickly, effectively and equitably by a more proactive approach. One of the arguments they use is that reductions in fertility in almost all poor countries have occured only in the presence of comprehensive family planning programmes. To assume that poor illiterate couples have no interest in controlling their family size is both patronizing and incorrect.

The principles underlying effective family planning programmes are straightforward and uncontroversial: a climate of public opinion needs to be created that is supportive of modern contraceptive use and the idea of smaller family sizes; knowledge of effective methods should be disseminated; a range of family planning services and products could be made accessible and affordable; and myths and misconceptions related to family planning must be adequately addressed. There is no blueprint for success. The key concerns are around the means of family planning promotion and service delivery. As in all preventive health strategies, context is the most important determinant of what combinations of interventions will work best, and priorities will evolve over time. The best family planning programmes have drawn extensively on local cultural knowledge and creativity to promote family planning, demonstrating the need for customization. The successful Bangladesh programme depended on a large cadre of female outreach workers going door to door to provide information, motivate clients and provide commodities. It also used mass media to stimulate a change in attitudes about family size. In the early phase of effective family planning programmes, the creation of legitimacy and awareness is crucial. As programmes mature, improvements to service quality, for instance, by phasing in new methods and making special efforts to reach underserved groups, are likely to become more important.

An initial priority is to legitimize the idea of modern family planning and smaller families. The first step is to create a broad coalition of support among key sectors of society, including religious, secular and traditional leaders, and professional groups. This strategy has proved important for sustained and effective programmes in many countries. Success in this depends more on political commitment and operational ability than on the availability of funds. Another important element is the use of the mass media. Evidence of its effectiveness in family planning is good. Not only do targeted messages, in didactic or dramatized form, raise awareness and prompt discussions between partners but they have also increased contraceptive use in both Asia and Africa, with favourable cost-effectiveness. Over and above the outcome of family planning messages, radio and television exposure also exerts a powerful effect on reproductive behaviour, presumably because of the transmission of new ideas and aspirations. Although spending on information and education has varied widely, evidence suggests that allocating 10–20 per cent of the country's family planning budget on this component makes good sense. Mobilization of support at the community level has been approached in various ways: women's credit groups in India and Bangladesh, mullahs in Iran and traditional village leadership committees in many African countries. Their effectiveness can be considerable, but community level efforts generally need skill, sensitivity and local cultural knowledge, qualities often absent in central government ministries.

As many as 85–90 per cent of couples will become pregnant within one year without contraception, and therefore even the least effective family planning method is much better than using nothing. Different contraceptive methods require different actions by users. The most effective methods typically in use are those that do not depend upon regular user action. Sterilization (both male and female), intrauterine devices and implants have 12-month failure rates of around 0.5 per cent or less when used perfectly, and with typical use the failure rate is less than 2 per cent. Injectable contraceptives (for instance Depo-Provera) have a similar figure of around 0.5 per cent with perfect use, but around 3 per cent with typical use. 'Perfect use' means that all the rules of the method are rigorously followed and (if applicable) the method is used at every act of intercourse. With perfect use the combined oral contraceptive also has a failure rate of less than 0.5 per cent but with typical use the failure rate is around 8 per cent, mainly due to inconsistent pill taking (poor adherence). The failure rates for perfect and typical use for male condoms are at 2 and 15 per cent, respectively, while withdrawal and periodic abstinence are even more difficult to adhere to, and hence have failure rates of around 25 per cent during typical use.

Specific methods used in different countries vary enormously. In Bangladesh, 43 per cent of contraceptive users rely on the pill; in neighbouring India, the corresponding figure is only 4 per cent while sterilization accounts for 75 per cent of all use. In many countries only one or two methods of contraception account for a large majority of all use. This failure to exploit the full range of contraceptive methods can be related to legislation against the use of specific methods, particularly sterilization, by government decisions to promote certain methods while ignoring or restricting access to others, and by biases of family planning providers. What is most familiar becomes most acceptable. When a couple discontinues contraception for method-related reasons, a rapid switch to a new method is essential to prevent unintended pregnancy. Limited choice of alternatives, and restricted access or unfamiliarity with other choices (on the part of both the user and the provider) can delay the uptake of a new method, increasing the risk of unintended pregnancy.

All contraceptive methods can reduce unintended pregnancy, but much potential is unrealized. Increasing the prevalence of use of any contraceptive method – even the least effective ones, encouraging switching from less effective to more effective methods, enhancing continuation of all reversible methods and boosting adherence to methods that depend on adherence for their effectiveness, all help. With the aim of raising the prevalence of use of any contraceptive method and the uptake of an alternative method after contraceptive discontinuation, a range of methods should be made available. In terms of cost-effectiveness of pregnancies prevented, sterilization and intrauterine devices are the best value, and the need to increase adherence becomes irrelevant. However, promotion of these methods has, in the past, clearly led to coercive methods in China, India and Vietnam. The most pressing priority for boosting prevalence of contraceptive use is in Africa, where sterilization is often not so appropriate since birth spacing is valued above limiting family size. In some African countries, injectable contraceptives have widespread acceptability, and the pill is commonly used. Promotion of these methods, together with condoms, via services with easy and reliable access, might offer the best chance of success.

Family planning programmes have made use of three main delivery systems: health facilities, commercial outlets and community-based approaches. In many countries, access to family planning methods was initially restricted to health facilities, under the strict control of medical practitioners. Often outdated eligibility criteria and other unnecessary constraints were used including the written consent of a husband, proof of marital status, parity, age, unwillingness to dispense more than one or two pill cycles and excessive revisit schedules. The limitations of these approaches were soon realized, and the success of many family planning programmes has been closely linked to dismantling administrative and medical barriers that impede quick, convenient and appropriate access to methods. Paramedical staff have been trained to insert intrauterine devices and provide injectable contraceptives to high clinical standards and community health workers, after a short training period, can dispense pills and refer women for clinical methods. Evidence also suggested that over-the-counter sales of contraceptive pills without prescription is justifiable.

Nevertheless, facility-based services remain the backbone of delivery systems in most countries, especially where surgical or clinical methods prevail. In most poor countries, more than 80 per cent of contraceptive sterilizations, intrauterine device insertions and administration of injectable contraceptives are done in hospitals and health centres. Poor quality of service is often the most important constraint on the uptake of family planning services. It is crucial to concentrate on fundamental issues such as the continuity of supplies, presence and competence of staff, treating patients with dignity and providing privacy. Since the 1994 Cairo conference, shifts have taken place towards a greater integration of services and towards broadening the scope of family planning clinics to address a wider range of reproductive health issues including reproductive tract infections, and HIV counselling and testing. Equally important is the addition of family planning to HIV/AIDS programmes in countries with severe generalized HIV epidemics. The prevention of unintended pregnancies in HIV-positive women is a more cost-effective way of reducing mother-to-child transmission than drug treatment. A 2008 World Health Organization review on linking reproductive health and HIV services found that integration leads to higher-quality and better-utilized services. Integration led to improved access to and uptake of services – including the use of modern contraceptives, increased HIV testing, and improvements in the overall quality of services. Countries with successful integration strategies include Ethiopia, Kenya, Lesotho and Uganda.

Commercial outlets such as pharmacies, shops and bazaars constitute the second most common way in which contraceptive methods are obtained. In many poor countries, advertising, logistics and product prices are subsidized through social marketing schemes typically run by international organizations. Partly in response to the threat of HIV/AIDS, the social marketing of condoms is now nearly universal in poor countries and is ideally suited for men and adolescents, for whom anonymous, quick access is important. In most countries, most condom users and a considerable proportion of pill-users obtain supplies from commercial sources. The third main mode of service delivery – outreach and community-based provision – complements social marketing. This has proved most useful in rural areas where access to other services is limited, when demand is fragile, and in places where women's mobility is constrained. A pre-condition for successful provision is that community health workers operate in their own communities, sharing the language and customs of their clients, and have credibility within their community. Other important lessons are that multipurpose community health workers are more effective and acceptable than those who provide only family planning, and that community involvement in the design of projects and the selection of the community health workers is essential.

How to revitalize the family planning agenda?

High fertility and rapid population growth represents a serious barrier to socioeconomic development. This is the message that needs to be conveyed to policy-makers. The threat to the achievement of nearly all Millennium Development Goals in many of the poorest countries, especially those in sub-Saharan Africa, posed by continued high birth rates and rapid population growth does not get enough attention; a 2005 74-page United Nations report on how to achieve the Millennium Development Goals mentions family planning in only two paragraphs. The priority owed to family planning as a development intervention must be stated explicitly. Evidence fully justifies this stance, although this viewpoint will arouse suspicions of a revival of the coercive tactics that were used in some Asian family planning programmes. Such suspicions must be addressed by emphasizing that no contradictions exist between a respect for reproductive rights and family planning promotion.

A further essential step is to press for greater recognition that the demographic circumstances in low- and middle-income countries are increasingly diverse and that prioritized actions must be tailored accordingly. It is clear that family planning need not be a top priority everywhere. Throughout much of Asia and Latin America, progress toward meeting family planning needs and population stabilization is well advanced. In these settings, the emphasis should be on improving the quality of services and meeting the needs of the poorest. However, in most of sub-Saharan Africa and some other countries including Afghanistan, Guatemala, Iraq, Laos, Pakistan and Syria with sustained high population growth and significant unmet need for contraception, family planning should return as a top priority. A delay in the onset of fertility decline in these countries where the populations are on course to double in size every 25–30 years, will have large implications for future population health, education and economic prospects.

Sources and suggestions for further reading

Kaddy's story and the findings of the research study on family planning and birth intervals in rural Gambia can be found in *Contingent Lives: Fertility, Time, and Aging in West Africa* by Caroline Bledsoe (Chicago: University of Chicago Press, 2002). Michael J. O'Dowd and Elliot Elias Philipp's chapter on 'Family Planning' in *'The History of Obstetrics and Gynaecology'* (New York: Parthenon, 1994, 457–480) was my main source of information on the history of family planning. To gain a better understanding of demographic transition and carrying capacity I made good use of the chapter 'Measures of health and disease in populations' by Adnan Hayder and Richard Morrow in *International Public Health Diseases, Programs, Systems and Policies* (eds Michael H. Merson, Robert E. Black and Anne J. Mills published by Jones & Bartlett in Sudbury, MA, 2005), as well as Tony McMichael's *Human Frontiers, Environments and Disease* (Cambridge: Cambridge University Press, 2001). The paper 'What is the demographic dividend?' by Ronald Lee and Andrew Mason (*Finance and Development*, 2006; 43: 3) explains the basics of the demographic dividend. John Cleland and colleagues' review paper on 'Family planning: The unfinished agenda' published in *The Lancet* in 2006

(368: 1810–1827) gives an excellent update on not only why family planning is still important but also on how to come to successful family planning programmes. The Demographic and Health Services website (www.measuredhs.com) provides a wealth of information on population, health, HIV and nutrition from over 75 countries, including comparative reports of contraceptive prevalence, and estimates of unmet need and the demand for family planning (last accessed 24 February 2010). Ruth Levine's text, *Case Studies in Global Health: Millions Saved* (Sudbury, MA: Jones and Bartlett, 2007), contains 20 very readable case studies of success stories in global health. Case 13 is dedicated to 'Reducing fertility in Bangladesh'.

6

Cervical cancer

Woman of Africa,
Sweeper,
Smearing floors and walls with cow dung and black soil,
Cook, ayah, the baby on your back,
Washer of dishes,
Planting, weeding, harvesting,
Storekeeper, builder,
Runner of errands, cart, lorry, donkey…,
Woman of Africa,
What are you not?

Okot P'Bitek, 1970

Maimuna

Maimuna, a 54-year-old mother of 7 and grandmother of 12, enters the outpatient clinic with a certain hesitation. She has travelled to Farafenni hospital from Bambali, situated on the North Bank of the river Gambia, 35km from Farafenni. Maimuna is accompanied by her daughter, Isatou, who speaks some English. Maimuna has complaints of weight loss, dizziness, increasing breathlessness even for the slightest physical activity, pains in the lower abdomen, and vaginal blood loss, although she is postmenopausal. She is not looking well, is cachectic, and is clinically severely anaemic. On internal pelvic examination I find a large inoperable tumour of the cervix that has invaded the surrounding tissues. The haemoglobin result confirms severe aneamia, and I admit Maimuna for blood transfusions, a biopsy from the tumour, and to begin pain medication, but I fear that her prognosis is bad and that we will not be able to do much for her.

Cancer

When you're diagnosed with cancer
Your choices are few
At first you really can't believe
What they plan to do to you

But there is no easy way to treat cancer
To beat it you need heavy-duty stuff
But you pray that they know to stop
When your body has had enough

Cancer treatment can be brutal
It may be hard to endure
But if you don't have the treatment
The cancer will kill you for sure

T. C. Rowe, 2001

Cancer develops when cells in one part of the body begin to grow out of control. Normally, cells grow, divide and die in an orderly fashion. During the early years of a person's life, normal cells divide more rapidly until adulthood. After that, cells in most parts of the body divide only to replace worn-out or dying cells or to repair injuries. Because cancer cells continue to grow and divide, they are different from normal cells. Instead of dying, they outlive normal cells and continue to form new abnormal cells. Cancer cells develop because of damage to DNA. Most of the time when DNA becomes damaged the body is able to repair it. In cancer cells, the damaged DNA is not repaired.

The origin of the word *cancer* is credited to Hippocrates (460–370 BC). He used the terms karcinos (Greek for crab), presumably because the pain resembles a crab's pinching. The oldest description of cancer (although the term was not used) and surgical treatment of cancer was discovered on papyrus rolls in Egypt and dates back to approximately 1600 BC. The papyrus described eight cases of tumours or ulcers of the breast that were treated by cauterization, with a tool called 'the fire drill'. However, the writing also says 'there is no treatment' for the disease. Treatment for cancer went through a slow process of development. There was a realization that there was no curative treatment once a cancer had spread and that intervention might be more harmful than no treatment at all.

In 1761, Giovanni Morgagni of Padua, Italy, was the first to perform autopsies routinely, and relate a patient's illness to pathologic findings after death. The 19th century saw the birth of scientific oncology, the study of cancer, with the discovery and use of the modern microscope. Morgagni had correlated the autopsy findings observed with the unaided eye with the clinical course of illness, while Rudolv Virchov (1821–1902) correlated the microscopic pathology, and provided the scientific basis for the modern pathologic study of cancer. This method not only allowed a better understanding of the damage cancer had done to a patient but also laid the foundation for the development of cancer surgery. This in combination with anaesthesia becoming available, allowed surgery to flourish and some great surgeons emerged who contributed to the modern art and science of cancer surgery. In 1889 Ernst Wertheim performed the first radical abdominal operation for the treatment of cervical cancer in Vienna, where he removed not only the cervix, but also the uterus and adnexes plus the surrounding and neighbouring lymph glands.

When Marie and Pierre Curie discovered radiation at the end of the 19th century, they stumbled upon the first effective non-surgical treatment. With radiation also came the first signs of multi-disciplinary approaches to cancer treatment. The era of cancer chemotherapy began in the 1940s with the discovery of nitrogen mustard, a chemical warfare agent, as an effective treatment for cancer, followed by folic acid antagonist drugs. Another breakthrough came in the 1960s with the realization that cancer chemotherapy should follow the strategy of antibiotic therapy for tuberculosis (see Chapter 3) with combinations of drugs, each with a different mechanism of action. The approach to patient treatment became more scientific with the introduction of staging and clinical trials. The staging became a routine process to determine the extent of a newly diagnosed cancer in a standardized manner, and is used to determine the appropriate treatment or combinations thereof. It also allows for the evaluation of treatment results, and to compare results from different types of treatment. Clinical trials comparing new treatments to standard treatments continue to contribute to a better understanding of treatment benefits and risks. Cancer treatment, with surgery, radiotherapy and chemotherapy as the primary modalities, has improved much over the last 50 years for many types of cancer in rich countries. In poor countries, cancer care is often unavailable or unaffordable for the poor in the context of very limited country health budgets and a high background level of acute and infectious diseases, and the persisting problem of high child and maternal mortality.

The 2006 second edition of the World Bank publication *Disease Control Priorities in Developing Countries*, in the chapter on Cancer Control, puts much emphasis on primary prevention to reduce or eliminate cancer-causing factors, and early detection and secondary prevention through population-based screening programmes to detect pre-cancer and cancer at a stage when curative treatment is possible. Unless cancer prevention and screening efforts effectively reduce the incidence of cancer, the number of new cases will increase from an estimated 10 million cases in 2000 to 15 million in 2020, 9 million of which would be in poor countries. By 2050, the cancer burden could reach 24 million cases per year worldwide, with 17 million occurring in poor countries. Despite the limitations of current data for poor countries, we know that the epidemiology of cancers in poor countries differs from those of rich countries in some important aspects. Rich countries often have relatively high rates of lung, colorectal, breast and prostate cancer because of the early onset of the tobacco epidemic, earlier exposure to occupational carcinogens, and the Western diet and lifestyle. In contrast, up to one-quarter of cancers in poor countries are associated with chronic infections. Liver cancer is often caused by hepatitis B infection, stomach cancer is associated with *Helicobacter pylori* infection, and cervical and oral cancers are associated with infection by certain types of human papillomavirus (HPV).

Cervical cancer

> *My prime interest was in the infectious origin of specific human cancers where epidemiology provided already some hints*
> Harald zur Hausen, 2008

Cervical cancer will develop in about 500,000 women this year worldwide, and it is the most common cancer of women in poor countries, which is where more than 80 per cent of all cases occur (Figure 6.1). The number of deaths from cervical cancer is estimated at 275,000 per year, and many of those who die are relatively young women as the disease is most commonly diagnosed among women in their forties. Not surprisingly mortality is highest in those countries least equipped to deal with the problem. Many women in poor countries present for care when a tumour is far advanced and inoperable, radiation is rarely available, and even palliative care is often of poor quality.

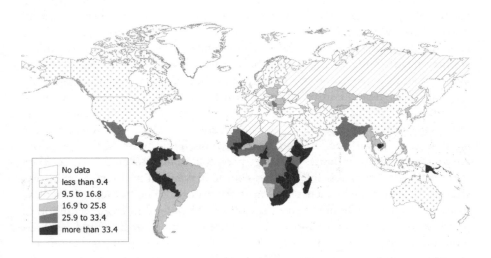

No data
less than 9.4
9.5 to 16.8
16.9 to 25.8
25.9 to 33.4
more than 33.4

Figure 6.1 *Map showing the global distribution of new cases of cervical cancer (age-standardized rate pr 100,000 female population per year)*

Source: *The GLOBOCAN 2002 data-base*, accessed at www.dep.larc.fr on 16 February 2010

Although cervical cancer is preventable with early diagnosis and treatment, in many poor countries it has been difficult to establish or maintain effective screening programmes. Initiation and maintenance of cytology-based screening programmes involving sexually active women every one to five years have had an important role in a large decline in cervical cancer incidence and mortality over the last 40–50 years in many rich countries. However, implementing such a programme in poor countries with inadequate health-service coverage, and low appreciation of preventative medicine has been problematic particularly in terms of accessing the population. Other hurdles to be overcome include increasing acceptability and availability of screening examinations, quality of specimen collection and evaluation, follow-up and treatment, the considerable cost and resource implications, and the demands of competing health needs.

Cervical cancer generally develops slowly over a period of 10–15 years. It is preceded by detectable and treatable pre-conditions in which certain cells in the cervix develop abnormal characteristics but are not yet cancerous. Broadly known as cervical dysplasia, these pre-cancerous abnormalities are classified according to severity. In 1713 Bernardo Ramazzini, an Italian doctor, had reported the virtual absence of cervical cancer in nuns and wondered whether this was in some way related to their celibate lifestyle. Only very recently, a causal link between HPV – the 'wart' virus, a sexually transmitted infection, and the development of cervical cancer was established, and it is estimated that over 99 per cent of such cancers worldwide contain HPV DNA. Harald zur Hausen, from Germany, received the 2008 Nobel Prize for demonstrating that HPV causes cervical cancer and was praised by the Nobel Committee for 'going against current dogma'. Commonly accepted risk factors for HPV and, therefore, for cervical cancer include a history of other sexually transmitted infections, early onset of sexual activity, having more than one sexual partner and/or a partner with more than one sexual partner. Other possible cervical cancer risk factors include early childbearing, high parity, tobacco use, use of oral contraceptives, genital schistosomiasis – a parasitic infection caused by the fluke *Schistosoma haematobium* – and nutritional factors.

Cervical cytology screening and alternatives

Cervical cytology is considered to be a very specific test for high-grade pre-cancerous lesions or cancer. However, even if the quality of collection and smearing of cells, fixation and staining of smears, and reporting by well-trained technicians is good, its sensitivity (that is the proportion of people with the disease who have a positive test result) is only 60 per cent. Frequent screening is needed to detect a missed high-grade pre-cancerous lesion during the subsequent rounds, and a high screening frequency has considerable cost and resource implications. Women with low-grade lesions are typically asked to return for a follow-up smear every six months so that progression or regression of the abnormality can be monitored. Women with a high-grade lesion are then evaluated using a colposcope, a special microscope that facilitates proper examination of the cervix and surrounding area, and undergo a biopsy to confirm diagnosis before treatment initiation. Colposcopy services in poor settings are often insufficient to meet the demand, partly due to a lack of trained colposcopists. Furthermore, colposcopes may not always function properly and are expensive and not easy to repair or replace. Follow-up is often problematic due to difficulties of specimen transportation, long delays between screening, diagnosis and treatment, inability to contact women with abnormal cytology results, and the difficulty of convincing women of the need for further evaluation and treatment.

Data on demand and acceptability of cervical cytology screening programmes are sparse. A South African anthropological study found that many women thought that a cervical smear was primarily diagnostic and not preventative. Coupled with a general perception that cancer of the 'womb' was inevitably fatal, this proved to be a powerful disincentive for many women to be screened. Few women in a Kenyan study were aware that early diagnosis and treatment of pre-cancerous lesions greatly improve the probability of a successful cure and prevention of cancer. Often limited information is provided to women, and as a result, misconceptions prevail. In addition there may be cultural barriers including fear of pelvic examinations, general inaccessibility and poor quality of health care services, including routine gynaecological care. It is not uncommon to find clinics in poor countries without trained personnel and laboratories, fresh water, electricity, slides, spatulas, and many of the other basic necessities for cytology-based screening programmes.

Several recent studies have demonstrated that direct visual inspection of the cervix with acetic acid or 'VIA' is a reliable, reasonably sensitive and cost-effective alternative to cytology screening. VIA requires a lower level of infrastructure and provides immediate results and the option for immediate treatment. However, the relatively low specificity (that is the proportion of people without disease who have a negative test result) is a problem that can result in overtreatment. Another unknown factor is how well VIA performs when genital schistosomiasis, that can simulate the features of (pre-)cancer, is prevalent. Standardized initial training and continuing education programmes including supervision and mechanisms for quality control will need to be developed if wide scale VIA screening is to be introduced, and there is also no research yet showing that VIA screening programmes reduce cervical cancer incidence and mortality.

HPV DNA testing is an alternative screening approach. HPV DNA testing of cervical samples obtained by health workers has the sensitivity for detection of high-grade lesions or cervical cancer that is equivalent or superior to that of cytology. But, HPV DNA testing is not (yet) cheap. A recent study from rural India, in which HPV testing was compared with cytological testing and VIA has shown very promising results. A single round of HPV testing significantly reduced the incidence of advanced cervical cancer and related mortality.

Screening methods should be combined with relatively simple, safe and effective, preferably outpatient, methods for the treatment of pre-cancer. In many poor countries, at present the only treatments available are cold-knife cone biopsy, whereby a cone-shaped sample of tissue is removed from the cervix, and hysterectomy, the surgical operation to remove the uterus and the cervix. Use of these methods not only results in overtreatment, both are associated with significant complications and side effects, and require major infrastructural support for anaesthesia, equipment and inpatient care, and consequently they are costly. For these reasons, loop electrosurgical excision procedure (LEEP) and cryotherapy are of interest for use in poor country settings due to their effectiveness, low incidence of side effects, low cost, lack of requirement for general anaesthesia and relative technical simplicity.

So what should be recommended for the screening and treatment of cervical (pre-)cancer in poor countries? The choice should be based on the comparative performance characteristics of the test, costs, technical requirements, level of development of laboratory infrastructure, capacity within the local health infrastructure and awareness and perceptions within the community. In very poor countries this might lead to a minimum package of a one-visit strategy of visual inspection with acetic acid and immediate cryotherapy treatment once in a life-time in the high risk age group of women between 35 and 50 years. This strategy ignores the low specificity of visual inspection and accepts overtreatment, but advocates of this approach will point out that cytological and colposcopic services are unlikely to become available in many resource-poor settings in the foreseeable future and that invasive cervical cancer represents a serious health problem for women that needs to be addressed immediately.

Vaccines

Given the long record of viral vaccines as a cost-effective approach to preventing life-threatening infections, an effective vaccine directed against the major cancer-causing HPV types could have a tremendous impact on the global cervical cancer burden, particularly if made available to poor countries. As we have seen, in many poor countries it has been difficult to establish and maintain effective screening and treatment programmes. On the other hand, these countries have, in many instances, developed comprehensive vaccination programmes against childhood illnesses such as polio, diphtheria, measles and tetanus, which, with appropriate adjustments, could prove instrumental in cervical cancer prevention.

Two vaccines have now been proven effective in preventing progression towards cervical cancer caused by HPV types 16 and 18, which account for 65–77 per cent of cancer cases worldwide. Merck's HPV vaccine, Gardasil, is very expensive, costing US$360 for the required three doses, and Glaxo Smith Kline's Cervarix is not much cheaper at about $335. Such prices are clearly not affordable for poor countries, where 80 per cent of cervical cancer cases occur. In addition, limited epidemiological data from the poor regions of the world that are available suggests that a much wider variety of HPV types, around 15, are involved in the pathogenesis of cervical cancer in poor countries. Longer follow-up is required to establish the degree of protection against these other cancer-causing HPV types, though preliminary findings are encouraging. Long-term monitoring is also necessary to determine the durability of protection and the need for additional immunization, the so-called 'booster'. The fact that HPV infection is a sexually transmitted infection (STI) may pose an obstacle to the acceptance of a preventative HPV vaccine, especially in countries where childhood vaccination against, for instance, polio is discouraged by fundamentalists who continue to spread false rumours about vaccines containing oestrogen to control births. Positioning an STI vaccine raises sensitive social issues, especially when it will be targeted at adolescents to ensure protection before the onset of sexual activity. Cheap, effective HPV vaccines are not yet available for poor people. If they become available and can be introduced successfully, the effect on cervical cancer reduction will not be felt for another 20–30 years, while the existing infections continue to progress to cancer. Screening will still be required.

Achieving broad coverage of adolescents for HPV vaccination, negotiating dramatic cuts in prices for poor populations, and securing financing will be challenging. It will need the involvement of global 'brokers' and donors such as the World Health Organization, the Global Alliance for Vaccines and Immunization (GAVI), the Bill and Melinda Gates Foundation, as well as the pharmaceutical industry. Given that with every 5-year delay in introducing vaccination and effective screening plus early treatment to poor countries, almost 1.5 million more women will die unnecessarily, one would hope that a concerted effort could be possible. The main message is that effective, affordable and appropriate solutions are within reach.

Palliative care

We ought to give those who are to leave life, the elderly, the terminally ill, those dying slowly of AIDS and cancer the same care and attention that we give to those who enter life – the newborn

Jan Stensward and David Clark, 2005

What happened to Maimuna? She received three blood transfusions during her admission that took away the dizziness and her breathlessness, she was given aspirin to reduce the pain which had only limited effect, and a biopsy was taken from the tumour site for histology diagnosis. After four days Maimuna wanted to go home and she was discharged with pain medication and given an appointment to come back to the outpatient clinic two weeks later. Unfortunately I could not prescribe Maimuna an oral opioid drug, as it was not available at the hospital pharmacy or in the private pharmacies. Maimuna did not come back for her appointment. One month later when I was visiting her village, I asked for Maimuna and was taken to her house. Isatou, her daughter was there and she told me about Maimuna's death three days earlier. Maimuna had refused to go back to the hospital as she thought it would not be of any help, she had increasingly felt tired and breathless as the irregular vaginal blood loss increased in frequency and quantity. But mostly it was the relentless pain that had denied Maimuna rest and sleep, and this had been most distressing to Maimuna and her family members who had provided care and support to her as well as others who came to visit her.

Worldwide, 57 million people die each year, and the vast majority of these in poor countries. Very little is known about the quality of care they receive at the end of their lives. The movement for improving the quality of care at the end of life is mostly focused on rich countries. Until it is considered as a global problem for public health and health systems, efforts to improve it will not have an impact on poor people.

It is estimated that there are hospices and palliative care services, either existing or under development, in about 100 countries around the world with between 7000 and 8000 palliative care initiatives including community-based teams, inpatient units and day-care centres. The distribution of these services is uneven and heavily weighted towards rich countries. Only approximately 6 per cent of all palliative care services are located in Africa and Asia, the regions where most of the world's population lives and dies. Little is known about the quality of care that people receive at the end of life in the majority of poor countries. However, available data show that the share of poor countries in the global consumption of morphine and other opioid drugs is only around 6 per cent, although these countries account for almost 80 per cent of the world's population. These figures illustrate the discrepancies in pain control between rich and poor countries and, possibly, the availability of palliative care that also involves contextually appropriate emotional, social and spiritual support to terminally ill people and their caregivers. Sufficient supplies of opioid drugs for use in palliative care are often not available in poor countries because of regulatory or pricing obstacles, ignorance or misconceptions.

Advocacy is needed to help raise awareness among government health departments as to what palliative care can offer and how even small changes in health policy can make a large difference in the quality of life of dying people. In particular, a review and adjustment of opioid control policies would remove one of the major barriers to palliative medicine. Hospice Africa in Uganda has demonstrated the feasibility of providing cheap oral morphine: at a cost of US$0.01 (1 cent) for a 10mg generic oral morphine sulphate tablet or morphine hydrochlorate solution made in the hospice pharmacy by the pharmacy dispenser, who has been authorized and is being monitored by the National Drug Authority. What is also needed is a broad knowledge base of palliative care and inclusion of palliative care training in undergraduate and postgraduate health professionals' training programmes, as well as continuing education programmes for established health care professionals. However, it is not only the health professionals who need to be educated but also the general public. Raising awareness about palliative care so that people know what options are available and are able to advocate for optimal care during a terminal illness, can help convince governments of the need to place palliative care on the national health agenda.

The silent burden of gynaecological disease in poor countries

There are no conditions of life to which a man cannot get accustomed, especially if he sees them accepted by everyone around him.

Leo Tolstoy, 1877

Two of the Millennium Development Goals directly address women's reproductive health: to reduce maternal mortality by 75 per cent and to halt and begin to reverse the spread of HIV/AIDS. While admirable, these goals ignore the prevalence of many treatable conditions causing death, disability and distress in women's lives. Accurate assessment of disease prevalence depends on accurate diagnosis, and this may be very difficult in resource-poor settings. Only a few comprehensive community-based studies in poor countries have sought to quantify the burden of gynaecological disease in order to influence policy. These studies have consistently shown a very high prevalence of previously unrecognized morbidity that places a heavy burden on women. The wide range of gynaecological diseases found included – next to cervical dysplasia – menstrual disorders, genital prolapse, pelvic masses, reproductive tract infections, infertility and related morbidity such as anaemia.

When I saw Maimuna at the outpatient department of Farafenni hospital in February 1999, we were in the middle of doing the first study in sub-Saharan Africa to estimate the burden of gynaecological disease at the community level. This study in rural Gambia revealed not only an enormous burden of disease but also that less than half of the women with reproductive health complaints had sought health care for their complaint. The most frequently reported reasons for not seeking health care were 'I didn't think it would help', 'too expensive', 'problem not serious enough', and 'afraid/embarrassed'. Some disorders were thought to be not worth reporting because they were considered normal for the individual, because they were widespread, or because there was a perception that nothing could be done. For example, women participating in semi-structured interviews on menstrual disorders were not aware of any treatments for irregularity or spotting.

The provision of services alone will not overcome the 'culture of silence' surrounding many of the reproductive health problems. Reproductive health care providers need to stimulate the demand for services at the same time as they are responding to this demand. There is also a need for a better understanding of behavioural factors, as well as gender and social aspects of health care. In primary health care clinics in Nairobi, Kenya, women's knowledge about health in general and sexually transmitted infections was poor, and a major gender difference was observed in a delay of health seeking for sexually transmitted infections (5 days for men versus 14 days for women). Although this difference in health seeking behaviour for sexually transmitted infections can be partly explained by the difference in signs and symptoms between men and women, there is more to it. The empowerment of women (and men) through education is a key factor in improving reproductive health. Not only are many reproductive health issues not subjects for public discussion, they are also seldom talked about even amongst peers. Reproductive choice and dignity will only be possible if prevalent notions harmful to reproductive health are questioned. Past neglect of reproductive health has often led to uninviting and inaccessible health services of poor quality. The combination of these factors represents an enormous challenge for under-resourced health services to provide appropriate care for women. The overriding challenge is to increase community knowledge about gynaecological diseases, their symptoms, prevention and treatment.

So where do we start? The arguments from welfare economics for the public funding of health care are persuasive when applied to reproductive health, and in many poor country settings it is difficult to envision serious reforms and improvement without increases in public-sector spending. However, communities themselves should assume some responsibility for women's health in ways that prioritize women's own perceptions and primary needs. Such programmes should be actively developed and evaluated for cost, benefit and sustainability. In addition, the social and financial empowerment of women is crucial. In many poor countries, women are often not in a position to attain and maintain their own health and well-being. This has to be changed if we are to address the large burden of gynaecological disease.

Sources and suggestions for further reading

For an historical perspective on cancer and cancer treatment, a good start is the section on the history of cancer on the website www.cancer.org (last accessed 20 January 2010). Dean T. Jamison and others' publication on *Disease Control Priorities in Developing Countries* (2nd edn, Washington: Oxford University Press and the World Bank, 2006), including the chapter on cancer control, is a comprehensive review of the cost-effectiveness of available interventions in the context of poor countries. For a relevant introduction on screening for cervical cancer see Lynnette Denny et al. 'Screening for cervical cancer in developing countries' (*Vaccine* 2006; 24: S3/71–77). The current state of knowledge of cervical cancer and human papillomavirus has been reviewed recently in Mark Schiffman and others' 'Human papillomavirus and cervical cancer' (*The Lancet* 2007; 370: 890–907). The issues around introducing HPV vaccines in poor countries have been discussed by Jan Agosti and Sue Goldi in 'Introducing HPV vaccine in developing countries – key challenges and issues (*New England Journal of Medicine* 2007; 356: 1908–1910) and Mark Kane et al. in 'HPV vaccine use in the developing world' (*Vaccine* 2006; 24: S3/132–139). Rengaswamy Sankaranarayanan led the team that evaluated the effectiveness of a single round of HPV testing, cytological testing or VIA in reducing the incidence of cervical cancer and associated mortality in women residing in rural India (*New England Journal of Medicine* 2009; 360: 1385–1394). Ruth Webster introduces the topic of palliative care in poor countries to public health professionals and health policy-makers, including making the case for the establishment of palliative care in 'Palliative care: A public health priority in developing countries' (*Journal of Public Health Policy* 2007; 28: 18–39), while the book by Michael Wright and David Clark, *Hospice and Palliative Care in Africa* (Oxford: Oxford University Press, 2006) provides a thorough background to the current challenges and opportunities for establishing palliative care in poor countries in Africa and elsewhere. The study that reports on the, partly silent, burden of gynaecological diseases in The Gambia can be found in G. Walraven et al. 'The burden of reproductive-organ disease in rural women in The Gambia, West Africa' (*The Lancet* 2001; 357: 1161–1167).

7

Water and sanitation

Water and sanitation is one of the primary drivers of public health. I often refer to it as 'Health 101', which means that once we can assure access to clean water and to adequate sanitation facilities for all people, irrespective of the difference in their living conditions, a huge battle against all kind of diseases has been won.

Lee Jong-wook, 2004

Neelum

Neelum has diarrhoea, she has had 5 bouts of watery non-bloody stool over the past 24 hours. Niloufer, Neelum's mother, tells us that it is her second episode of diarrhoea since the last full moon. Neelum is six months old, and is still being breastfed but Niloufer had started giving her two spoons of water after breastfeeding soon after birth. This amount of water had been increased gradually, and now Neelum is getting about one and a half cups of water four times a day. Neelum is irritable, has sunken eyes and a skin pinch goes back slowly – signs of minor, but not severe dehydration. On the advice of the community health worker Niloufer has already started giving Neelum oral rehydration fluids, which she drinks eagerly. Neelum is not very sick; she is not vomiting, has no fever and on clinical examination no other abnormalities are found. But her growth is faltering as her weight gain has only been 100 grams over the last three months.

In the mountain village in Northern Pakistan where Neelum lives with her family, water has to be fetched from the unprotected village pond and only a small minority of the households has a toilet within the homestead. Others, including the members of Niloufer's family use the open fields and surroundings. During our visit, Neelum's two-year-old sister defecates in the compound, upon completion of which Niloufer promptly removes the faeces with a shovel and throws it on the street and the girl is washed with water stored in a clay pitcher. There is no organized sanitation or solid waste management in the village. Solid waste is thrown on garbage heaps in the streets, which is then spread by animals, rain and wind. Wastewater in Neelum's compound is collected in a pit which flows to the street where no drainage system exists. Niloufer knows that boiling water can help prevent diarrhoea, but limited firewood prohibits her from doing so. From talking to Niloufer, her husband and other villagers it becomes clear that there is very limited awareness of the role of safe water, adequate sanitation and hygiene in the prevention of diarrhoea.

A child under five years of age in Pakistan is estimated to suffer from an average five episodes of diarrhoea per year. Diarrhoea is the leading cause of childhood death in Pakistan. Several factors are likely to contribute to high diarrhoea morbidity and mortality rates, including poverty, female illiteracy, low status of women and young children, chronic undernutrition, poor water supply and sanitation, poor hygiene practices and inadequate health services. In the 1980s, the Pakistan government, supported by UNICEF and the World Health Organization, launched programmes to reduce the large burden of childhood diarrhoea deaths, mainly by promoting oral rehydration therapy (ORT). However, death from diarrhoea still persists as a major problem.

Safe water

> Sir,
>
> *May we be and beseech your protection and power. We are Sir, as it may be, living in a Wilderness, so far as the rest of London knows anything of us, or as the rich and great people care about. We live in muck and filth. We have got no privacy, no dust bins, no drains, no water-supplies, and no drain or sewer in the whole place. The Sewer Company, in Greek St., Soho Square, all great, rich powerful men take no notice whatsoever of our complaints. The Stench of a Gulley-hole is disgusting. We all of us suffer, and numbers are ill, and if the Cholera comes Lord help us.*
>
> Anonymous Letter to the Editor, *The Times*, 1849

In August 1854 cholera cases began to appear in Soho, Central London. A drastic increase in the week ending 2 September led London's pioneering anaesthetist John Snow, who had gained experience with cholera during the 1831 epidemic in Newcastle upon Tyne, to investigate all 93 local cholera deaths. Snow painstakingly enumerated every facet of the local houses, inns and shops, and water consumption patterns of their permanent and temporary inhabitants. He concluded that the local water supply was contaminated, for nearly all victims used water from the Broad Street Pump. At a nearby prison, conditions were far filthier, but deaths were few – it had its own well. On 7 September John Snow requested the local Board of Guardians to disconnect the pump. Sceptical but desperate, they agreed. The handle of the pump was removed, and the number of cases plummeted, and Snow had confirmation of his theory that cholera was caused by the contamination of drinking water, and that it was a 'water-borne' disease.

The closing of the Broad Street pump has become an iconic moment in the birth of public health, but at the time Snow was ignored. In 1855, he gave his views to a House of Commons Select Committee: cholera, he maintained, was not contagious and neither a poison in the ambient air but rather was water-borne. He advocated massive improvements in the drainage and sewage, a call that played some part in the investment by the London authorities in new main drainage and sewage systems. After 'the great stink' in the summer of 1858 that caused Parliament to break off its proceedings, an ambitious scheme was started for the mains drainage of London, based on proposals from Joseph Bazalgette, the Metropolitan Chief Engineer. This was completed in 1875. London's water was increasingly drawn from the higher reaches of the river Thames and from the Lea Valley, and filter beds were developed. Only after another epidemic in 1866 was John Snow's evidence of water-borne infection given belated recognition. It took until 1883 for Robert Koch, the godfather of bacteriology and also the discoverer of the organism that causes tuberculosis, to identify the cholera bacillus in India and show that it was conveyed in water polluted by the faeces of victims.

I have been in a 'Snow' situation, where I had to advise the local authorities to stop the use of unprotected water sources three times, twice in Tanzania and once in The Gambia. In all instances (twice it concerned outbreaks of cholera, once of dysentery) the authorities and communities fully cooperated, and again in all three situations the number of cases plummeted. But each of the outbreaks had by then already been the cause of several completely unnecessary deaths.

Water-borne and water-related diseases

Truly 'water-borne' transmission occurs when the pathogen or disease-causing agent is in the water and is drunk by a person who then becomes infected. Potentially water-borne diseases include the classic infections like cholera and typhoid, but also a wide range of other diseases, such as infectious hepatitis, diarrhoeas and dysenteries. The term 'water-borne disease' has been greatly misused so that it has become almost synonymous with all water-related disease. Water-related diseases also include other groupings such as 'water-washed diseases', where a key consideration is an inadequate volume of water for washing people, clothes, food, utensils and so on. Diseases in this group include scabies and trachoma. Other classifications of water-related diseases are 'water-based' and 'water-related vector' diseases. A water-based disease is one in which the pathogen spends a part of its life cycle in a water snail or other aquatic animal. All these infections are due to infection by parasitic worms (helminths) which depend on aquatic intermediate hosts to complete their life cycles. Examples include diseases such as schistosomiasis and guinea worm. Water-related vector diseases are spread by insects which either breed in water or bite near water. Malaria, yellow fever, dengue and onchocerciasis (river blindness) are transmitted by insects which breed in water while African trypanosomiasis (sleeping sickness) in West and Central Africa is transmitted by the tsetse fly which bites near water.

Another source of misunderstanding arises from the implication in the label 'water-borne', that water is the disease's only means of transmission. This preoccupation has its origins in the dramatic water-borne epidemics of cholera and typhoid in London and European towns in the 19th century, which were blamed on poor urban water supplies with inadequate treatment facilities. It should be noted that water-borne diseases can also be transmitted by any route which permits faecal material to pass into the mouth. Thus diarrhoeas may be spread by indirect faecal–oral routes, for instance via contaminated food, soiled clothes, door latches, taps and drinking pots unintentionally touched with faecal material. Small children who play in the dust and dirt of a household compound and constantly put their fingers in their own and other's mouth are particularly at risk. Next to the protection of household drinking water against faecal contamination, good hygiene, especially hand-washing, is key to stopping the transmission of diarrhoeal disease. In addition, fly control during periods of high fly densities has been shown to be an effective measure to reduce diarrhoea incidence.

Whereas the prevention of water-borne diseases often requires improvements in water quality, water-washed diseases can be stopped by improvements in availability – the quantity – of water used for hygiene. Protecting the water supply may also affect water-based and water-related vector transmission. For example, if it reduces the need to enter water where there are schistosome-infected snails, or if a more reliable water supply averts the need for keeping water-storage vessels in which dengue vectors breed.

The haves and the have nots in water

A slum dweller in Nairobi or Dar es Salaam, forced to rely on private water vendors, pays 5 to 7 times more for a litre of water than an average North American citizen.

Anna Tibaijuka, 2004

The strange paradox of community water supply in poor countries is that, in one sense, everyone has a water supply while in another sense, many people have not. Water is essential for life and all human communities must have some kind of water source. It may be dirty, it may be inadequate in volume and it may be several hours' walk away but, nevertheless, some water must be available. However, if we apply any reasonable criterion of adequacy – in terms of the quantity, quality and availability of water – then many people in poor countries do not have an adequate supply. What constitutes a satisfactory water supply to some communities leaves others, even in poor countries, considering themselves underserved. In much of rural Africa, a hand pump 500 metres from the household is a luxury. In Asia, urban planners would consider a community served if there were sufficient stand posts on the street corner; however, if the water only flows for a few hours per week, producing lengthy night time queues, the residents may regard this situation as a lack of service and opt to buy water expensively from water vendors. As these examples illustrate, water supply is not a single, well-designed intervention, such as immunization, but can be provided at various levels of service with varying benefits and differing costs.

Reasonable access has been internationally defined as the availability of at least 20 litres per person per day from a source within 1 kilometre of the user's dwelling. Whether the water supply is 'safe' is difficult for communities and responders in population surveys to determine, and therefore the indicator of 'improved' water supply has been introduced. Respondents in surveys can indicate the type of technology involved, and improved water supplies can be expected to provide water of better quality and with greater convenience than traditional not improved sources. Household connection, public standpipe, borehole, protected well and spring, and rainwater collection are considered as 'improved' water supply. An unprotected well, river or spring, vendor-obtained water and water supply via a tanker-truck are considered 'unimproved'. There are an estimated 880 million people without access to improved drinking water resources (this figure was 1.2 billion in 1990), and of these, an estimated 84 per cent live in rural areas. A lack of progress in reducing the numbers of people without access to water is of particular concern in sub-Saharan Africa (see also Figure 7.1 which shows the percentage of population with access to an improved water source per country). The benefits to health are not

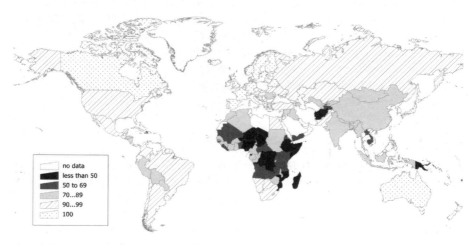

Figure 7.1 *Map showing the global distribution of access to improved water (%)*

Source: Millenium Development Goals Indicators. The official United Nations site for the MDG indicators at mdgs.un.org/unsd/mdg (accessed on 17 February 2010)

normally foremost in the minds of those provided with new water supplies, it is the time and energy saved which is the most obvious benefit when water is made available closer to the household. In rural areas in poor countries it remains commonplace for women and children to spend at least one hour a day collecting water.

Sifat

Sifat has been asked by his school teacher to go and see the doctor. Sifat, who is 11 years old, is feeling progressively tired and is increasingly out of breath. He stopped playing cricket in the school yard, and now must stop several times when he climbs the hill to go home after school. Both he and his teacher have observed that he has difficulty concentrating during his classes, and his test marks have gone down over the last few months. He complains of dizziness and palpitations. On examination, there is marked pallor of his conjunctivae as well as his palms which are whitish in colour. He has some pitting oedema of his feet and ankles. Sifat has a fast heartbeat with what is called a bounding pulse. The heart sounds are loud. The combination of auscultation and percussion of his chest shows a displacement of the heart's apex and therefore a likely enlargement of the heart. The liver is enlarged and tender to palpation, but smooth. Sifat is admitted in the local health centre with the provisional diagnosis of 'high cardiac output' heart failure complicating severe anaemia, and investigations are carried out to determine the cause and severity of the anaemia. He has a haemoglobin of 5.3 grams per decilitre, confirming the clinical diagnosis of severe anaemia, and the blood film shows that his red blood cells are hypochromic (which means that they have a exaggerated central pallor) and microcytic (abnormally small) – pointing in the direction of iron deficiency anaemia. His stool is dark in colour, and is positive on testing for occult blood. Microscopy of Sifat's stool sample shows hookworm eggs in very high quantity (equivalent to 27,000 eggs per gram of faeces). The diagnosis is made of severe hookworm anaemia, and Sifat is given an intravenous transfusion of packed red blood cells, oral iron therapy is started, and he is also given deworming tablets (mebendazole). He is likely to recover quickly and be able to do well again in school and return to his beloved cricket.

When a health care provider in a poor country receives the result of a patient's blood smear and detects that the red blood cells are hypochromic and microcytic, he or she will immediately recognize iron deficiency anaemia, which might very well become the diagnostic label for the patient. This is correct, but the implications go beyond simple iron medication. A deeper understanding of this patient may reveal, as was the case with Sifat, that the patient is suffering from hookworm anaemia, which led to blood loss via the intestinal mucosa and explains the subsequent iron deficiency anaemia. Contamination with hookworm is often – as was the case for Sifat – related to the absence and/or inadequacy of latrines. The construction and maintenance of latrines has proven to be the most powerful measure to reduce the burden of this kind of anaemia. So, while an inward-looking laboratory-oriented health care provider might be content to establish the diagnosis 'iron-deficiency anaemia', a more outward-looking health care provider might prefer the (much more operational) diagnosis 'latrine-deficiency anaemia', a concept hitherto unheard of in conventional medical textbooks.

Many schools for health professionals in poor countries copy their undergraduate and postgraduate medical, nursing and allied health sciences education from rich countries, where maternal and child mortality is low, where the burden of poverty-related infectious diseases is low, and life expectancy high. In many poor countries, the result is that health professional students, interns and registrars are trained in sophisticated high-tech methods rather than in getting a basic understanding of engineering methods for the improvement of community health. We need both inward-looking and outward-looking providers, and more holistic comprehensive training in health sciences. A significant community health component is of great importance if we want to create graduates who can identify and devote themselves to research and efforts to reduce early mortality and the large burden of disease in poor countries.

Adequate sanitation

Too often, the 'sanitation' component of 'water and sanitation services' is referred to only in passing, as if clean water alone will solve the personal environmental crisis confronting the world's poorest citizens

Willem-Alexander, Prince of Orange, 2008

While John Snow is the hero of the Broad Street water pump, there was another investigator. The Reverend Whitehead, curate of a nearby parish, and like John Snow a member of the Cholera Inquiry Committee, also carried out a house-to-house investigation in the area, confining his inquiry to Broad Street. Whitehead delved deeper than Snow into the mystery of how and why the well had become infected. At number 40 Broad Street, Reverend Whitehead discovered that there had been an earlier case of a cholera-like disease, and that excreta from this patient had been thrown into a cesspool very close to the well. A surveyor was then called. He found the brickwork of drain and cesspool highly defective, with a steady percolation of fluid matter from the privy into the well. Whitehead thus not only confirmed Snow's water-borne disease theory, but pinpointed the main cause: inadequate sanitation. Although safe drinking water took on the majority share in much later efforts to address 'water-borne' diseases in poor countries, the Victorians themselves were very focused on sanitation and sewerage. Their efforts to impose 'cleanliness' on the poor had all the characteristics of a moral crusade.

Industrialized poverty on such a scale was a new phenomenon, and the 'barnyard conditions amid stench and filth' which characterized the crowded tenements and alleyways in which poverty stricken people lived were horrendous.

As we have seen, improvements in excreta disposal can have differing degrees of influence on faecal–oral diseases. Since most of the water-related diseases (and several others not related to water) are caused by pathogens transmitted in human faeces, these can be controlled, at least partly, by improvements in water supply. These and the other excreta-related diseases are also affected by the improvement in excreta disposal, ranging from the construction of or improvement in toilets, to the choice of methods for transport, treatment, and final disposal or re-use of excreta. One category in the other excreta-related diseases are those caused by soil-transmitted helminths. This category contains several species of parasitic worm including hookworm, ascaris (roundworm) and trichuris (whipworm) whose eggs are passed in faeces. They are not immediately infective, but require a period of development in favourable conditions, usually in moist soil. Since the eggs are not immediately infective, personal cleanliness has little effect on their transmission, but any kind of latrine which helps to avoid faecal contamination of the floor, yard or fields will limit transmission. However, if a latrine is poorly maintained and the floor becomes soiled, it can become a focus of transmission.

Diarrhoeal diseases, mostly associated with a lack of safe potable water, not enough water, inadequate sanitation, poor hygiene and combinations thereof, account for an estimated two million deaths per year, and of these a vast majority are in children under five years old, almost all in poor countries. And the mortality figures represent only a tip of the illness iceberg: tens of millions of children suffer repeated bouts of diarrhoea during their early years. The spread of oral rehydration therapy, in which UNICEF and the World Health Organization have been closely involved for the past 30 years, is important in tackling one of diarrhoea's most lethal symptoms: dehydration and electrolyte imbalance caused by the loss of gut fluids. But some diarrhoeal infections such as bacterial dysentery cannot be managed with oral rehydration therapy only. Such infections also require antibiotics. In the end, there is only one way to reduce the toll of childhood diarrhoeal disease and death, by preventing as many infections as possible in the first place. In June 2009, the World Health Organization recommended that a rotavirus vaccine be introduced in national immunization programmes. Rotavirus, also transmitted via the faecal–oral route, is thought to be the leading single cause of severe diarrhoea in infants and young children, and the vaccine was found to significantly reduce severe diarrhoea episodes in studies in Latin America, South Africa and Malawi. In a statement on the recommendation to give rotavirus vaccine to all children, the World Health Organization also said, 'because there are other causes of diarrhoea, it is also important to improve water quality, hygiene and sanitation'.

Soil-transmitted helminth infections

Diarrhoeas are the most important excreta-related problem, but soil-transmitted helminths, whose eggs mature in faeces and enter the body through the feet or mouth, also do great damage. The presence of faeces in compounds, pathways, fields and other places where 'open defecation' is the norm puts adults and children – especially if they run around barefoot – at risk. Of particular importance are the roundworms, whipworms and hookworms which infect hundreds of millions of people. They produce a wide range of symptoms including diarrhoea, abdominal pain, general malaise and weakness. Roundworms, whipworms and hookworms are often considered together because it is common for a single individual, especially a child living in a poor country, to be chronically infected with all three worms. Such children often experience undernutrition, growth stunting, intellectual retardation, and cognitive and educational deficits. Studies have highlighted the profound negative effect of soil-transmitted helminth infection on school performance and attendance, and economic productivity. Hookworms cause chronic intestinal blood loss that results in – as we have seen in the case of Sifat – anaemia.

Anti-helminthic drug treatment ('deworming') is aimed at reducing disease by decreasing the worm burden. Repeated chemotherapy at regular intervals in high-risk groups can ensure that the infection-levels are kept low and results in immediate improvement in child health and development. Obstacles that diminish the effectiveness of periodic deworming are the low efficacy of single-dose drugs for the treatment of hookworm and trichuris, high rates of post-treatment re-infection for soil-transmitted helminths in areas with high endemicity, and diminished effect with frequent and repeated use, possibly because of antihelminth resistance. Sanitation is the only definitive intervention to eliminate soil-transmitted helminth infections, but to be effective it should cover a high percentage of the population. The importance of sanitation in controlling disease in general was stressed in a poll carried out in 2006 by the *British Medical Journal*. More than 11,000 readers chose 'the sanitary revolution' as the most important medical milestone since 1840, when the *British Medical Journal* was first published, followed by the discovery of antibiotics and the development of anaesthesia.

The haves and the have nots in sanitation

More than 1.2 billion people worldwide gained access to improved sanitation between 1990 and 2004. However, even with this progress, there are an estimated 2.5 billion people (this was 2.7 billion in 1990, the world population growth did not help) – 40 per cent of the world's citizens – without access to improved sanitation. To halve the proportion of people without access to safe drinking water and basic sanitation by 2015 (the target of Millennium Development Goal 7) will be especially challenging for sanitation. Most notably, South Asia and sub-Saharan Africa are 'off-track'(see Figure 7.2 for improved sanitation access per country). Providing sanitation in rural areas is the most difficult challenge: it is projected that about 1.7 billion rural people will remain without improved sanitary facilities in 2015. Similar to water, for sanitation the term 'improved' has also been introduced. It includes connection to a public sewer, connection to a septic system, a pour-flush latrine, a ventilated improved pit latrine as well as a simple pit latrine. Sanitation solutions that are not considered as 'improved' are public or shared latrine, open pit latrine and bucket latrine.

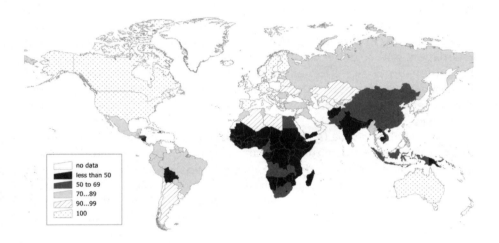

Figure 7.2 *Map showing the global distribution of access to improved sanitation (%)*

Source: *Millenium Development Goals Indicators.* The official United Nations site for the MDG indicators at mdgs.un.org/unsd/mdg (accessed on 17 February 2010)

The impact of not improved or poor sanitation extends beyond health. We often fail to appreciate how undignified and personally distressing it is to have no decent place to 'go'. Women, especially in rural areas, were in the past able to go out under the cover of darkness to a nearby area, set aside specially for the purpose, with bushes and trees to protect their privacy. Nowadays, the bushes and trees are often gone, there are considerable distances to walk, and girls and women risk being attacked if they venture out so far at night. Where schools do not provide proper toilets for children, and particularly for girls, their educational prospects suffer. Faced with a lack of girl-friendly facilities, many parents withdraw their daughters from school when they reach adolescence. Clean, safe and dignified toilet and hand-washing facilities in schools can help ensure that girls get the education they need and deserve. When they get education, the whole community benefits – it raises economic productivity, reduces poverty, lowers infant and maternal mortality, and helps improve nutritional status and health.

Economic, social and environmental benefits from improved water supply and sanitation

Good water and sanitation services, accompanied by hygiene promotion, confer many benefits. Conversely, the costs of not providing water and sanitation services can be significant in terms of lost opportunity and inverse impacts on economic and social development, and environmental sustainability. Achieving the water and sanitation related Millennium Development Goal targets underpins the achievement of several other Millennium Development Goals such as those on poverty alleviation, health, hunger, education and gender equality. Providing improved water and sanitation services enables children such as Neelum and Sifat to avoid illness and to attend school. An integrated intervention using appropriate technologies that pays attention to water supply, water quality, drainage, sanitation and school- and community-based hygiene education in villages in Northern Pakistan in the area where Neelum and Sifat live, resulted in children living in intervention villages having a 33 per cent lower chance of having diarrhoea than children living in non-intervention or control villages. Improved water supply frees up the time of women and children involved in carrying water. Sufficient water of adequate quality is also essential for the productivity of various business sectors – food and beverages, manufacturing, mining, energy, tourism, etc. Sanitation plays a critical part in water-related benefits, as it influences the quality of the water that returns to the ecosystem.

To put in place basic improved water supplies (with standpipe, bore hole, dug well or rainwater harvesting) costs somewhere between US$17 and $55 per capita. Similarly, the construction of a simple pit latrine, a ventilated improved pit latrine or a pour-flush latrine costs between $26 and $91 per capita, while septic tank installation ($104–160) and sewer connection ($120–160) are more expensive. The relatively large variations in costs are related to the local circumstances and conditions, as well as the population density. A recent World Health Organization report estimates that $18 billion will be needed annually to extend existing infrastructure to achieve the water and sanitation related Millennium Development Goal targets, roughly doubling current spending. And even if these targets are achieved, millions of people – the 'other' 50 per cent – will still not have access to improved water and sanitation.

The World Health Organization also estimates that each dollar invested in water supply and sanitation generates $4–12 in health benefits alone, depending on the type of water and sanitation service. This is a substantial return for society as a whole, but it does not accrue directly to policy-makers, investors and the community at large. The results so far of the General Assembly of the United Nations proclaimed 'Decade for Action: Water for Life' (2005–2015) and the 'International Year of Sanitation' (2008), that were meant to achieve a greater focus on water and sanitation related issues at all levels, are (too) limited. Greater efforts are needed to document and communicate the economic, social and environmental benefits of investing in water supply and sanitation, and in water resources management, particularly to economy and finance ministers, and to donors. More effective communication with the public is also needed to explain the benefits that they receive, and how their contributions are being utilized. Most poor countries face a gap between the levels and quality of water and sanitation services they would like to provide and what they can afford. Closing this gap requires good information and analysis, discussion among stakeholders, and appropriate measures to reduce the demand for, and increase the supply of, finance.

Aid, in the form of grants and loans, for water supply and sanitation has been rising since 2001, after a decline in the 1990s. Over the period 2002–2006, aid for water and sanitation doubled in real terms, and the total was around $6.2 billion in 2006. The share of water supply and sanitation in total aid also increased from 2002 to 2006, rising from 6 per cent to 9 per cent. However, there are concerns about the regional and country distribution of aid to water and sanitation. Much of it flows to countries that already have relatively good access to water supply and sanitation, or have enjoyed a favoured relationship with a particular donor. For example, Albania, Costa Rica, Iraq, Jordan, Lebanon and Malaysia all received at least $13 per capita of water and sanitation aid, while Angola, Central African Republic, Republic of Congo, Somalia and Togo received less than $0.5 per capita. Overall the poorest countries received just one-quarter of the total aid for water supply and sanitation, other low-income countries a further quarter, and middle-income countries about half. The share of aid to the water and sanitation sector in sub-Saharan Africa has recently declined from 27 per cent to 22 per cent.

Expanding access to improved water and sanitation is a moral and ethical imperative. Safe and sufficient water and adequate sanitation is of crucial importance to the preservation of human health, especially among children. If the Millennium Development Goal target for water and sanitation were met, the health-related costs avoided could reach an estimated $7.3 billion per year, and the annual global value of adult working days gained as a result of less illness would be almost $750 million. Improvements in water, sanitation and hygiene contribute to improved health, generate savings for households and national health budgets, and contribute to poor households' economies through reduced costs and loss of time. Saving time may enable productive activity and school attendance, especially for girls. Investment in water and sanitation makes economic sound sense. Extending water supply and sanitation services to poor households everywhere would also make important contributions to promoting the globally shared values of dignity, equity, compassion and solidarity. Appreciation of the linkages between water, sanitation, hygiene, health and quality of life are not new. If the case is clear and the effectiveness of actions well known, what more is needed? It is a priority to which the global health community needs to give greater attention.

Sources and suggestions for further reading

Sandy Cairncross and Richard Feachem's *Environmental Health Engineering in the Tropics. An Introductory Text* (London: John Wiley and Sons, 1993) remains a very informative book for anyone who wants to acquire an understanding of environmental health issues and engineering solutions in poor countries. Maggie Black and Ben Fawcett's *The Last Taboo: Opening the Door on the Global Sanitation Crisis* (London: Earthscan, 2008) tells the world's untold stories of sanitation, including the history of human waste, but provides as well practical information and guidance to increase the proportion of the population with access to sanitation. The article by Jeffrey Bethony and others on 'Soil-transmitted helminth infections: Ascariasis, trichuriasis, and hookworm' in *The Lancet* (2006; 367: 1521–1532) provides a good review on this subject. The study by D. Nanan and others entitled 'Evaluation of a water, sanitation, and hygiene education intervention on diarrhoea in northern Pakistan' in the *Bulletin of the World Health Organization* (2003; 81: 160–165) reports on the effectiveness of an integrated intervention on children having diarrhoea referred to in the text. 'Impact of fly control on childhood diarrhoea in Pakistan: Community-randomised trail' was reported in *The Lancet* by Desmond Chavasse and others (1999; 353: 22–25). The findings of the poll in which readers chose the sanitary revolution as the greatest medical advance since 1840 can be found in the *British Medical Journal* (2007; 334: 111). To study the health, economic, social and environmental benefits from improved water supply and sanitation I made good use of chapter 41 'Water supply, sanitation, and hygiene promotion' written by Sandy Cairncross and Vivian Valdmanis in *Disease Control Priorities in Developing Countries* (a co-publication of Oxford University Press and the World Bank, 2nd edn, 2006) edited by Dean Jamison and others; the article 'Focusing on improved water and sanitation for health' by Jamie Bartram and colleagues that appeared in *The Lancet* (2005; 365: 810–812); as well as *Managing Water for All: An OECD Perspective on Pricing and Financing* (Paris: OECD, 2009), and a 'problem paper' by Guy Hutton on *Unsafe Water and Lack of Sanitation* that he wrote for the Copenhagen consensus centre (downloaded from the www.copenhagenconsensus.com website on 12 November 2009).

8
Neglected tropical diseases

Neglected tropical diseases are 'the low-hanging fruit'
interventions because success has been achieved in their control
with strategies that are cost-effective, deliverable, effective, and
which provide 'beyond-disease-specific' benefits

David Molyneux, 2010

Ousman

It is February 1998, mid-afternoon and a hot dry wind blows through the small village of Farato in rural Gambia. Most people are inside their huts or have sought a shady place under a tree or elsewhere. We visit Alhaji's compound. Alhaji is 68 years old, he is blind and has been blind for more than 20 years. His corneas are completely opaque. We examine the three children in the compound. Alhaji's grandson Ousman – he is four years old – has our special attention as he has a very unclean face with significant nasal discharge. Eversion of his eyelids and examination of the superior tarsal conjunctiva, with the aid of a magnifying glass and a torch, reveal the presence of numerous discrete follicles. Ousman has active trachoma. He not only gets a sweet for sitting still and being good during the examination, we will also give him an oral dose of the antibiotic azithromycin, to be repeated annually for a number of years, to treat his eye disease, as well as advising the whole family on face and hand washing.

Trachoma

Such is its character that the man who suffers from it burrows in
darkness, and lives out his life (the disease is generally incurable)
in dread of light. Any brightness sears the nerves of the brain like
molten metal.

Anonymous, *Time*, 1924

Trachoma is a chronic eye infection that usually begins in childhood, sometimes with redness (pinkeye), itching and pain. The disease and blindness result from recurrent and multiple infections with *Chlamydia trachomatis*, which occur over a period of 10–20 years. During this time, recurrent infections lead to scarring of the eyelids. When the scarred eyelids turn inward, the lashes scratch the surface of the eyeball, leading to inflammation and scarring of the cornea and ultimately blindness. These later stages are known as trichiasis.

Recorded knowledge of trachoma dates back as far as 1550 BC, with descriptions appearing in the Egyptian Ebers papyrus. Ancient Greek physicians were also familiar with the disease, and Galen described the rough lining of the upper eyelid that is symptomatic of repeated infections. Scholars believe the biblical passage about Leban's eldest daughter, which states 'Leah was tender eyed', is describing trachoma. It is thought that St Paul, Cicero, Horace and Galileo all had trachoma. When Napoleon began his quest into Egypt in 1789, he not only had to fight the Egyptian army, but also blinding eye diseases that would incapacitate thousands of his soldiers. Military or Egyptian ophthalmia, as the disease was called, infected 3000 of Napoleon's troops in a period of ten weeks, blinding many. Although military ophthalmia was viewed as a single disease, the affliction was actually a combination of several eye infections, including *Haemophilus influenza* conjunctivitis, gonococcal conjunctivitis and trachoma. Most likely the gonococcal infections were responsible for the rapid onset of blindness.

When Napoleon's troops withdrew from Egypt they spread ophthalmia, including trachoma across Europe, where trachoma had been present only sporadically. British troops and soldiers of other European nationalities were also infected with trachoma as a result of their military campaigns in Egypt. A common belief was that only soldiers who had served in Egypt could have trachoma. However, as soldiers and civilians who had never been to Egypt began contracting the disease, the contagious nature of trachoma became understood. Trachoma became widespread, and many of the eye hospitals founded in Europe in the 19th century were established specifically for the treatment of trachoma. In 1810, the British government appointed an expert committee to investigate trachoma. The team recommended that infected people should be isolated and cleanliness was emphasized. Treatments also included removal of granulations on the inner eyelid and various eyewashes. The British government created special schools where infected children were isolated. Strict hygiene measures were reinforced according to the expert committee guidelines. The schools succeeded in stopping transmission from infected to healthy children and helping infected children to recover from infection without progressing to blindness. The fact that nurses and staff at the schools did not become infected gave further support to recognizing that hygiene was key to trachoma control.

At the end of the 19th century and beginning of the 20th century, many migrants left Europe and set out for a new life in America. Anxiety about diseases being brought into the country by immigrants led to legislation being passed in 1891 by the US Congress stating, 'that the following classes of aliens shall be excluded from admission into the United States ... persons suffering from a loathsome or a dangerous contagious disease'. The concern about trachoma was so great that in 1897, trachoma was the first contagious disease classified as loathsome or dangerous by the US government. It became policy that immigrants to the US were routinely screened for trachoma on arrival at Ellis Island, New York, and sent back to their country of origin if they had it – more than 36,000 were declined access and especially those who were poor. As living standards improved in industrialized countries in the 20th century, trachoma disappeared; the last trachoma isolation hospital in the UK closed in 1947.

Chlamydial inclusions were first described in conjunctival epithelial cells from patients with trachoma in 1907, and in 1954 Chlamydia trachomatis was isolated and cultured by T'ang and colleagues in China. The organism was then used to inoculate a blind volunteer at London's Institute of Ophthalmology, and the subsequent development of symptoms of trachoma in the volunteer confirmed that Chlamydia trachomatis was indeed the infective organism responsible for the disease. For a large part of the 20th century, the agent of trachoma was thought to be a virus because it was so small and could only be grown within living cells. By the 1970s however, Chlamydia trachomatis was acknowledged as a bacterium because it became clear that it possesses both DNA and RNA and it is susceptible to antibiotics. In 1937, scientists discovered that sulphanilamide is effective in treating trachoma. However, many people were allergic to sulpha antibiotics and experienced a severe skin reaction, so efforts continued to find an alternative treatment. In the 1950s oral and topical tetracyclines were found to be effective, and, since oral or systematic tetracyclines carry serious side effects, topical tetracyclines became the treatment of choice. Tetracycline ointment, to be applied twice daily for six weeks, was the recommended regime for active trachoma until the 1990s when azithromycin, which is effective in one oral dose, became the preferred treatment for trachoma.

In 1998 a World Health Organization Assembly resolution called for member states to take steps to eliminate blinding trachoma by 2020 using the SAFE strategy: Surgery of late stage disease, Antibiotics for acute disease, and improved Facial and Environmental hygiene – meaning face washing and improved access to water and sanitation. Trachoma is usually described as a 'water-washed' disease because it is caused by dirt and germs getting into children's eyes, and washing the face is an important means of prevention. However, adequate sanitation can also help prevent trachoma. More than 70 per cent of the incidence of the infection has been shown to be caused by flies, mainly of the species Musca sorbens, commonly known as the bazaar fly, which prefers to breed in scattered human faeces. In studies in the Farafenni area in The Gambia, pit latrines were shown to reduce the population of these flies by depriving them of their breeding sites, which in turn produced a reduction in active trachoma and diarrhoeal disease.

The International Trachoma Initiative, founded in 1998 by the pharmaceutical company Pfizer and the Edna McConnel Clark Foundation, now supports the SAFE strategy in 18 countries. These countries had the majority of the global burden of active trachoma disease and a large proportion of the backlog of trachoma-related eye saving surgery. Since 1999 this initiative has been able to facilitate more than 400,000 eye saving surgeries and over 100 million azithromycin treatments have been administered. Morocco was the first country using the SAFE strategy to eliminate blinding trachoma, followed by other countries including, most recently, Ghana. Other countries, such as The Gambia, Mauritania and Vietnam continue to progress in the reduction of the active disease and the elimination of trachoma might be achieved within a few years. Ousman was checked and treated on an annual basis as part of a mass campaign for several years, and active disease has vanished from him, his family and his community. Although there are still an estimated 40 million people who suffer from active trachoma infection in 56 countries (see Figure 8.1), and over 8.2 million people living with advanced trachoma (trichiasis) and facing visual impairment or blindness unless treated surgically, the progress against blinding trachoma attained by a number of countries highlights the feasibility of the SAFE strategy and the possibility of the global elimination of the disease. In a period of around ten years, some of the world's poorest countries have planned and implemented successful programmes and demonstrated measurable short-term impact.

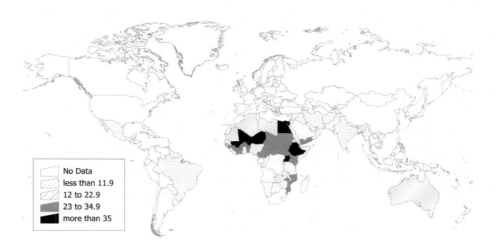

Figure 8.1 *Map showing the global distribution of active trachoma in children under 10 years of age (%)*

Source: World Health Organization. Prevention of avoidable blindness and visual impairment programme at www.who.int/blindness/data_maps/en (last accessed on 23 February 2010)

Leprosy

Now the leper on whom the sore is, his clothes shall be torn and his head bare; and he shall cover his moustache, and cry, 'Unclean! Unclean!' He shall be unclean. All the days he has the sore he shall be unclean. He is unclean, and he shall dwell alone; his dwelling shall be outside the camp.

Leviticus 13, c.1440 BC

Leprosy's physical symptoms – scaly flesh, mutilated fingers and toes and bone degeneration, made it seem a living death and led to deeply punitive attitudes. Leprosy was highly stigmatized. Authorized by the Old Testament Levitical decrees, leper laws were strict in medieval Europe. Leprosy sufferers were forbidden all normal social contacts and became targets of shocking rites of exclusion. Leprosy was thought to be a hereditary disease, a curse or a punishment from God. Leprosy sufferers could not marry, they were forced to wear special clothing, and ring the 'Lazarus' bells to warn others that they were close. Even in modern times, leprosy treatment has often occurred in separate hospitals and live-in colonies called leprosariums because of fear of infection and the stigma of the disease. This is very well described in Victoria Hislop's bestselling novel *The Island* which gives a detailed account of life on Spinalonga, the former leper colony north of Crete in Greece. Gerhard Hendrik Armauer Hansen of Norway in 1873 identified under the microscope the germ, *Mycobacterium leprae*, that causes leprosy, and therefore proved that it was not hereditary, nor a curse or punishment for sin. In 1941, Promine, a sulfone drug, was introduced as a treatment for leprosy, but unfortunately many painful injections were required. Dapsone pills became the treatment of choice in the 1950s, but sadly and relatively quickly, *Mycobacterium leprae* began developing dapsone resistance. The first successful multi-drug treatment regimen was developed in the 1970s.

Now, leprosy has been reduced as a public health concern and is endemic in only nine of what was previously a list of over 100 countries: Angola, Brazil, Central African Republic, Democratic Republic of Congo, India, Madagascar, Mozambique, Nepal and Tanzania. The global registered prevalence of leprosy has been reduced to 224,000 cases. Since 1985 some 14.5 million people have been cured through multi-drug therapy. The numbers of new cases per year has fallen dramatically, at an average rate of 20 per cent per year. The new multi-drug treatment regimen to cure leprosy is donated by the pharmaceutical company Novartis. The expectation is that the global elimination of the disease – similar to trachoma – is achievable within a generation.

Neglected tropical diseases are poverty promoting diseases

These neglected tropical diseases affect the poorest populations in the world, causing unnecessary suffering and reducing productivity and development. By working together to ensure there is synergy in our interventions, we can achieve greater coverage more rapidly, thereby improving their health and helping to alleviate poverty.

Jacob Kumaresan, 2006

Trachoma and leprosy control are making good headway to becoming success stories, and both diseases are included in a group of diseases that in general does not get the attention it deserves: the neglected tropical diseases. Millennium Development Goal 6 refers to combating HIV/AIDS, malaria and 'other diseases', which fuelled the desire to recognize these other diseases and create advocacy constituencies that emphasize the need for their recognition. The fraction of the global population infected with HIV (30 million of the bottom billion) raises issues of equity, as David Molyneux, one of the leaders in the battle against the neglected tropical diseases, stated. This is in view of 'the burden of diseases on the 960 million without HIV or those who have survived malaria but are now exposed to other debilitating infections of poverty'. There is still no standard definition of neglected tropical diseases, but one can say that there are two approaches to defining these diseases. The first approach emphasizes neglect as the defining characteristic, whereas the second concentrates on the diseases' shared features and their effect on poverty and development. Recent definitions draw more attention to the second approach. The neglected tropical diseases have several things in common. They affect the poorest of the poor, but rarely affect the well off. The group includes the bacterial infections trachoma, leprosy and Buruli ulcer and the infections caused by the soil-transmitted helminths hookworm, *Ascaris* and *Trichuris*. This group also includes other, mainly water-related, helminth infections such as guinea worm, onchocerciasis, schistosomiasis and lymphatic filariasis, as well as the vector-borne protozoan infections leishmaniasis, African trypanosomiasis and Chagas' disease. As shown in Table 8.1, approximately 1 billion poor people suffer from *Ascaris*, *Trichuris* or hookworm infections, while roughly 200 million people suffer from schistosomiasis, 120 million from lymphatic filariasis, 40 million from trachoma, and 37 million from onchocerciasis. Common features of the so-called neglected tropical diseases include high endemicity in rural areas and in the urban slums of poor countries, relatively low mortality but an ability to impair childhood growth, intellectual development and education, as well as worker productivity. You could say that these neglected diseases are 'poverty-promoting conditions'.

The high prevalence of the neglected tropical diseases is often not appreciated by policy-makers, sometimes even including government officials from countries where neglected tropical diseases are endemic. An important

Table 8.1 *The 13 major neglected tropical diseases listed by control strategy*

Neglected tropical disease	Status	Control strategy
Diseases controllable by mass drug administration (MDA)		MDA control
Soil transmitted helminths: Hookworm, Ascaris, Trichuris	Over 1 billion infected annually (sub-Saharan Africa, South-East Asia, Latin America)	Annual treatment with albendazole or mebedazole, improved water and sanitation
Schistosomiasis	200 million infected – mostly in Africa	Treatment with praziquantel, improved water supply and sanitation
Lymphatic filariasis (elephantiasis)	120 million infected in Africa and South Asia, 43 million suffer from hydrocele, lymphoedema and other evidence of severe lymphatic filariasis disease	Six annual MDA with albendazole + ivermectin (in onchocerciasis endemic countries) or albendazole + diethylcarbamazine (in non-onchocerciasis endemic countries)
Trachoma	40 million with active disease, 8.2 million visually impaired – eliminated from some countries, incl. Morocco and Ghana	Annual treatment with azithromycin, as part of the 'SAFE' strategy
Onchocerciasis (river blindness)	37 million infections in Africa	Annual treatment with ivermectin
Diseases controllable by environmental measures		Provision of filtered water
Guinea worm	Close to eradication	Individual case finding and case containment, surveillance, improved safe water provision and filtration, vector control of water fleas
Diseases requiring individual treatment		Case control
Chagas disease	8–9 million infected. Limited distribution in South America – a disease of poor housing	Control of the bed bugs which carry the disease
Cutaneous leishmaniasis	1.5 million new cases annually, with a total of 12 million people infected. 90% of cutaneous leishmaniasis cases occur in Afghanistan, Brazil, Iran, Peru, Saudi Arabia and Syria.	Early diagnosis and prompt treatment, control of sand fly populations through residual insecticide spraying, use of insecticide-impregnated bed nets (vector control is rarely used)
Visceral leishmaniasis	500,000 cases per year. 90% of all visceral leishmaniasis cases occur in Bangladesh, Brazil, India, Nepal and Sudan; fatal if untreated	Case finding and treatment

Table 8.1 *continued*

Neglected tropical disease	Status	Control strategy
African Trypanosomiasis	0.3 million infected. Narrow distribution in Africa dictated by the tsetse fly distribution	Case finding and treatment, vector control
Buruli ulcer	Global prevalence 50,000. Endemic in 30 countries in the Americas, Africa and South East Asia	Early diagnosis, treatment with antibiotics or surgery
Leprosy	Close to elimination	Case finding followed by multiple drug therapy

reason for the lack of awareness about these conditions is that the neglected tropical diseases are seldom found in those parts of the capital cities where the government officials work and live. They truly are, as Peter Hotez, another leader in the battle against neglected tropical diseases, calls them 'forgotten diseases afflicting forgotten people'. Another characteristic is that conflict, civil unrest and health service collapse are intimately related to neglected tropical diseases. Refugees, migrants and ethnic minorities in conflict with central governments are additionally vulnerable to these diseases. A few examples include leishmaniasis in Afghanistan; guinea worm in Sudan; lymphatic filariasis in Myanmar; onchocerciasis and human tryponosomiasis in Angola, Democratic Republic of Congo and Sudan. Many of the neglected tropical diseases are disfiguring and stigmatizing, their characteristics are described in the Bible and other ancient texts, affirming that they have affected humans for millennia. But, as they affect the poorest of the poor, there are few or no commercial markets for the drugs and vaccines needed to treat neglected tropical diseases. The pharmacopoeia for many of these diseases has remained essentially unchanged (or has dwindled) since the middle of the 20th century.

The burden of disease resulting from the neglected tropical diseases is substantial, with an estimated 530,000 deaths annually, and many more people who suffer from early disability. More than 400,000 of these deaths are caused by five diseases: schistosomiasis, hookworm, ascariasis, leishmaniasis and African trypanosomiasis. Perhaps even more significant than the mortal burden is the amount of impairment, often described in the literature as the years of active life lost that result from premature disability. The health impact of neglected tropical diseases is one element in terms of their adverse impact on development. Because of their chronic and disabling features, neglected tropical diseases also produce important educational and socioeconomic consequences that keep affected populations poor. Chronic hookworm infection in childhood dramatically reduces future wage-earning capacity, and lymphatic filariasis erodes a significant component of India's gross national product. Although it is typically painless and rarely results in death, the ulcer of Buruli disease can have severe consequences for the patient as well as the health system given the costs of surgery and care that have to be devoted to those suffering Buruli ulcers in advanced cases. For instance, tissue destruction can lead to infection of the underlying bone (known as osteomyelitis) and sometimes this necessitates limb amputation. Also, if lesions occur near joints such as the knee or elbow, the subsequent healing can result in contractures that prevent the use of the limb.

In a typical West or Central African community affected by onchocerciasis or 'river blindness', sight loss commonly begins to occur in the fourth decade of life. Thus, in the hardest-hit African communities, individuals who normally are parents and heads of households – the breadwinners – are rendered blind. Frequently, they are guided by their child or grandchild who therefore has to stop attending school. They themselves cannot contribute appreciatively to the economic well-being of their farming communities. The socio-economic consequences of this scenario are devastating. When river blindness reaches epidemic proportions, there are too few people to tend the fields, resulting in food shortages and the abandonment of homelands in otherwise fertile river valleys. When subsistence farmers are forced to migrate further from rivers where the infecting black flies breed to regions with poor soils, entire village communities can be thrown into poverty.

Neglected tropical diseases do not occur in isolation. In many poor countries at least five neglected tropical diseases occur in the same area. The three soil-transmitted helminths and schistosomiasis exhibit considerable geographical overlap with lymphatic filariasis, onchocerciasis and trachoma. This allows for an integrated programme for either the control or even elimination of these seven neglected tropical diseases using a combination of four drugs – albendazole, ivermectin, azithromycin and praziquantel. Three of these drugs are currently donated by pharmaceutical companies, while the fourth (praziquantel) is available at a relatively low cost. Each of the drugs has overlapping specificity so that multiple pathogens are concurrently targeted. In addition, the four-drug regimen also targets other infections, including scabies and several bacterial respiratory tract infections.

HIV/AIDS, tuberculosis and malaria can be considered as the 'big three' devastating communicable diseases, attracting by far the most attention. Adding to their complexity is the geographical and epidemiological overlay with neglected tropical diseases in many poor countries, especially sub-Saharan Africa. Helminths are the most common parasites found in HIV-, tuberculosis- and malaria-infected populations, especially the three major soil-transmitted helminths, as well as the two major schistosomes and the filariae. There is substantial co-morbidity when the neglected tropical diseases are 'superimposed' on HIV/AIDS, tuberculosis and malaria, with anaemia probably being the most important consequence of multi-parasitism and multiple infectious causes. Co-infection with the neglected tropical diseases also adversely affects the natural history and progression of the 'big three'.

Helminth co-infections might increase susceptibility to malaria and HIV, and accelerate the progression of HIV disease. Research in Zimbabwe has shown that women with urinary schistosomiasis, which causes irreversible lesions in the genital area and can therefore create a lasting entry point for HIV, had a three-fold increased risk of having HIV. Giving praziquantel to school age and adolescent girls in urinary schistosomiasis infected areas might be a cost-effective way to protect them from both schistosomiasis morbidity and HIV infection. There is also some evidence that helminth infections, especially hookworm and schistosomiasis might adversely affect the outcome of pulmonary tuberculosis or the progression to active tuberculosis. Integrating neglected tropical diseases control into programmes addressing HIV, tuberculosis and malaria has the potential for large collateral benefits. The community-based health care systems created to deliver neglected disease drugs could be well suited to administering antiretrovirals, directly observing adherence to tuberculosis therapy, improving access to antimalarials and increasing the use of insecticide treated bed nets. At the same time, neglected tropical diseases control would benefit from control efforts for the big three. For example, insecticide treated bed nets used in malaria control are highly effective at interrupting the transmission of lymphatic filariasis, and many antiretrovirals would be expected to reduce the impact of leishmaniasis.

Control of neglected tropical diseases

It has been estimated that for a cost of about US$200 million annually, approximately 500 million poor people ($0.40 per patient) could receive preventative treatment in a four-drug integrated package. Such a programme would have to be maintaind for a period of 5–7 years to effect a sustained global assault on the seven major tropical diseases which can be treated with the four-drug package. The integrated approach provides cost savings of almost 50 per cent compared to 'piece-meal' individual disease efforts. To further increase efficiencies, several public–private partnerships have together created an alliance, the Global Network for Neglected Tropical Diseases, to begin a global campaign for integrated control in 56 countries where at least five important neglected tropical diseases co-exist (see Figure 8.2). As a scaling up of integrated control moves forward, a number of questions need to be answered, including issues of secure drug supply, compliance, drug interactions and emerging drug resistance.

Of the different drugs contained in the integrated package, the agents albendazole and its alternative mebendazole stand out as drugs that could induce resistance. Both albendazole and mebandole belong to the benzimidazole class of drugs. Other drugs in this group are widely used to de-worm livestock of their soil-transmitted helminths. For decades, livestock producers in tropical and subtropical regions have relied heavily on frequent periodic treatments with benzimidazole antihelminths to ensure that their animals harbour low worm burdens throughout the year. Today, however,

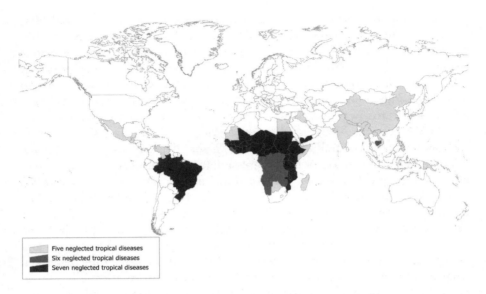

Figure 8.2 *Map showing overlap and global distribution of the seven most common neglected tropical diseases*

Source: Hotez, P. *Forgotten People, Forgotton Diseases.* HSM Press, Washington, D.C., 2008

resistance to benzimidazole is widespread in many regions and this resistance now thwarts livestock production in several regions in the world. There are some observations which suggest the possibility that benzimidazole resistance has occurred among human helminth parasites, especially hookworms as well as filariae after scaled-up use of alebendazole and ivermectin combinations. There is also evidence of a lack of efficacy of ivermectin in Ghana that needs further investigation.

The occurrence, fortunately so far only in sporadic instances, of drug resistance in the treatment of some neglected tropical diseases should not, according to Peter Hotez, deter us from aggressively working to deploy the rapid impact integrated packages in poor countries. He argues that resistance to helminths does not evolve as rapidly as it does for bacterial or viral pathogens, but that it is important to put in place the tools and mechanisms for monitoring the emergence of drug resistance with urgency. At the same time, we need to continue research and development efforts for a new pipeline of drugs for neglected tropical diseases. As new drugs are developed, they could be introduced into integrated drug packages when necessary. However, a major obstacle for the development of treatments for neglected tropical diseases is the absence of a viable commercial market and therefore the absence of incentive for pharmaceutical companies to embark on drug development projects for these diseases. Anti-helminth drugs were mainly developed for veterinary use where profits for the pharmaceutical companies made drug development worthwhile. These companies have made money from them and were therefore ready to consider donations or a low cost supply. Although the major pharmaceutical companies have been willing to donate selected products free of charge in order to combat neglected tropical diseases in poor countries, it is difficult for a publicly held company responsible to shareholders to take the next step and commit precious resources toward extensive research into and development of new products for these diseases. Yet, without donations for neglected diseases the afflicted populations could never afford such products. The Global Forum for Health Research has coined the term '10/90' to describe the observation that only 10 per cent of global funding for medical research and development is spent on problems that affect the poorest 90 per cent of people in poor countries. The sufferers of the neglected tropical diseases are obviously major victims of this phenomenon.

Despite some track record of developing new drugs for neglected tropical diseases, it is unrealistic to think there will be a significant improvement in research and development capacity for new agents if we rely on multinational drug companies alone. What is needed are 'product development partnerships' or PDPs. These PDPs have been described as 'public-health-driven not-for-profit organizations that drive neglected-disease drug development in conjunction with industry groups', and several of these partnerships are now in place – some of which are supported by the Bill and Melinda Gates Foundation. Initiatives are also in place, albeit still mostly at the basic research stage, to develop vaccines for neglected tropical diseases, including schistosomiasis, leishmaniasis, hookworm, Chlamydia (both for trachoma and genital Chlamydia infections that can also cause neonatal pneumonia through infection via the birth channel), Buruli ulcer and Chagas disease.

At the same time, if we accept the principle of striving to get existing rapid-impact integrated drug packages to the people who urgently need them, it is vital that economic analyses of these integrated packages are undertaken. Studies of the economic rates of return of large-scale and successful neglected tropical disease control and elimination programmes, such as onchocerciasis control in West Africa, guinea worm eradication, lymphatic filariasis and schistosomiasis control in Egypt and China, and Chagas disease control in South America, have shown very good returns. It is conceivable that an equal or greater return could be achieved with a rapid impact package targeting multiple neglected tropical diseases. However, as explained in Chapter 7, the concept of integration should be expanded beyond chemotherapy and include access to improved water and sanitation, as well as education and communication strategies to address the root socio-economic, ecological and behavioural causes of neglected tropical diseases.

Sources and suggestions for further reading

The paper 'Trachoma through history' by Kathrine Schlosser and accessed on the International Trachoma Initiative website (www.trachoma.org) was an important source for the description and history of trachoma, while for the history of leprosy my main source of information was (again) Roy Porter's *The Greatest Benefit to Mankind* (London: N.W. Norton, 1997). For the description of the burden of trachoma, clinical features and solutions to the problem, including the possibility of elimination I consulted, amongst others, papers by David Mabey and others (*The Lancet* 2003; 362: 223–229); Jeffrey Mecaskey and colleagues (*Lancet Infectious Diseases* 2003; 3: 728–734); and Matthew Burton and David Mabey (*PLoS Neglected Tropical Diseases* 2009; 3: e460). The paper reporting on the association between pit latrines and active trachoma can also be found in *The Lancet* (2004; 363: 1093–1098: Paul Emerson et al. 'Role of flies and provision of latrines in trachoma control: Cluster-randomized trial'). Victoria Hislop's *The Island* (London: Headline Review) was first published in 2005. Peter Hotez, David Molyneux, Alan Fenwick and Lorenzo Savioli are the outstanding individuals in the neglected tropical diseases movement. They are determined to transform the neglected tropical diseases into 'former' tropical diseases, at least in the sense of these diseases being brought decisively under control if not fully eliminated. They are also the authors of the article 'Rescuing the bottom billion through control of neglected tropical diseases' (*The Lancet* 2009; 373: 1570–1575). Other sources used include another paper by David Molyneux: '"Neglected" diseases but unrecognised successes – challenges and opportunities for infectious disease control' (*The Lancet* 2004; 364: 380–383); the article by Peter Hotez et al. 'Incorporating a rapid-impact package for neglected tropical diseases with programs for HIV/AIDS, tuberculosis, and malaria' (*Public Library of Sciences Medicine* 2006: 3; e102); as well as Peter Hotez' book *Forgotten People, Forgotten Diseases: The Neglected Tropical Diseases and their Impact on Global Health and Development* (Washington, DC: ASM Press, 2008) which is an excellent primer into the world of the neglected tropical diseases. For an entry-point to a better understanding of the co-endemicity of schistosomiasis and HIV see 'HIV/AIDS, schistosomiasis, and girls' (Kari Stoever et al., *The Lancet* 2009; 373: 2025–2026). In addition, in January 2010 *The Lancet* ran a Special Series on the neglected tropical diseases, while there is also – since 2007 – an open-access quality journal publishing peer-reviewed research solely dedicated to the neglected tropical diseases (see www.plosntds.org). Evidence of the efficacy of the control of soil-transmitted helminths through de-worming in Zanzibar is described by M. Albonico et al. (*Bulletin of the World Health Organization* 2003; 81: 343–352). To tackle schistosomiasis mass drug administration with praziquantel has been successful, especially in Morocco and Puerto Rico, where the disease is close to elimination (see A. Fenwick et al. *Advances in Parasitology* 2006; 61: 567–622). K. Ichimori et al. describe lymphatic filariasis elimination from the Pacific region (*Trends in Parasitology* 2007; 23: 36–40), while the impressive success of the guinea worm eradication programme is described by E. Ruiz-Tiben and D. Hopkins (*Advances in Parasitology* 2006; 61: 275–309). Descriptions of the modern history of programmes for onchocerciasis control can be found in B. Boatin and F. Richard (*Advances in Parasitology* 2006; 61:

349–394). Morocco became the first middle-income country to successfully interrupt the transmission of trachoma through the SAFE strategy, and an account of this success can be found in Case 10 of Ruth Levine's *Case Studies in Global Health: Millions Saved* (Sudbury, MA: Jones and Bartlett, 2007). The control of Chagas disease in South America is described by Y. Yamagata and J. Nakagawa (*Advances in Parasitology* 2006; 61: 129–165). The two major approaches for the control of human African tryponosomiasis are described by E. Fèvre E et al. (*Advances in Parasitology* 2006; 61: 168–221), while control of leishmaniasis (both cutaneous and visceral) remains difficult due to its complex epidemiology, lack of early diagnostic tools and the high cost of the medicines that need to be injected (J. Alvar et al. *Advances in Parasitology* 2006; 61: 223–274). New approaches to treat and prevent Buruli ulcer have been reported by P. Johnson et al. (*PLoS Medicine* 2005; 2: e108), while A. Rinaldi provides a review of the global campaign to eliminate leprosy (*PLoS Medicine* 2005; 2: e341).

9

Undernutrition

Nutrition belongs to the very basic facts of life. We are what we eat. A child becomes what it has eaten. Could it be that the cause for overlooking the significance of the nutritional status is that it is too apparent?

H. A. C. P. Oomen, 1953

Hassan

Hassan looks at me with his big eyes in his old man's wrinkled face. Hassan is 10 months old, is 58 cm long and weighs 3.9 kg. He had been admitted two days earlier at Bamyan Hospital in Central Afghanistan with cough, high fever and fast breathing, and crepitations were found on auscultation at the base of both lungs. Today Hassan is better, the fever is down, the signs and symptoms of pneumonia have disappeared and the antibiotics course started at admission might very well have contributed to the improvement. However, this is Hassan's third admission to the hospital over a period of four months; once previously for pneumonia and once for severe watery diarrhoea and dehydration. What worries me most is Hassan's lack of weight gain – his 'road to health' chart where his monthly weights have been plotted against age is completely flat. Hassan was, at 2400 grams, a low-birth weight baby after a normal gestational period, but he had caught up and had gained weight well until six months of age. Fatima, Hassan's mother, tells us that Hassan is her third child in a period of four years, and that she is now five months pregnant again. Hassan was exclusively breastfed for only six weeks, as early complementary feeding with sheep's milk is customary in her community. When Hassan was seven months old she stopped breastfeeding him completely on the advice of a health worker when the health worker found out that Fatima was pregnant, and Fatima was given some formula milk by this health worker. Fatima mainly feeds Hassan the local staple foods – rice, potatoes and bread made out of wheat, but there are no vegetables, except onions, nor fruits now in the months after the winter. Fatima and her husband cannot afford to buy many food items, and Hassan rarely eats eggs or fish or meat.

The famous Buddhas of Bamyan were not the only thing destroyed in the quarter century of civil conflict in Afghanistan. Undernutrition killed and disabled many children in Afghanistan, and prevented many others from reaching their full intellectual and productive potential. And this undernutrition problem continues to today.

Diseases of deficiency

The notion that disease could be due to a lack of something involved a new paradigm. 'Disease is so generally associated with positive agents – the parasite, the toxin, the *materies morbid*', noted a report in 1919, 'that the thought of a pathologist turns naturally to such positive associations and seems to believe with difficulty in causation prefixed by a minus sign'. Among the disorders to which this novel concept seemed applicable was marasmus, afflicting infants in impoverished areas and characterized by muscle-wasting, fat loss and low body weight. Another was kwashiorkor (from the Ga language of coastal Ghana, translated literally as 'first-second' and meaning a disease suffered by a child displaced from the breast when a younger sibling comes), mainly found in sub-Saharan Africa, typified by oedema, anorexia, enlarged liver, diarrhoea and lethargy. In 1755 the French physician Gaspar Casal had published an account of pellagra, then a new disease in Spain. Characterized by dermatitis ('a horrible crust, dry, scabby ... crossed with cracks') and a cause of diarrhoea, dementia and premature death, it flared up every spring. Casal noted that its victims were poor; had maize as their staple food, and they had very little meat or milk. Joseph Goldberger (1874–1929), of the US Public Health Service, noticed that in orphanages and mental asylums where inmates developed pellagra, the staff (naturally on better rations) escaped. If eggs and milk were added to inmates' diet, the disease diminished. After dermatitis appeared in convict volunteers put on a maize-meal diet, Goldberger concluded that the disease was due to lack of (as then unknown) dietary factors.

Beriberi was common in the rice cultures of Asia. Singhalese for 'I cannot', beriberi is characterized by weakness in the legs, hands and arms. Weakening of the cardiac muscles leads to heart failure. Hindsight shows that beriberi became especially severe in the late 19th century in South-East Asia because the large populations labouring on plantations and working in mines survived largely on milled rice, from which the husks had been removed. Christiaan Eijkman, director of a research laboratory at Batavia (Jakarta), first observed in the 1890s that the hospital chickens developed polyneuritis when they were fed the white rice given to patients, rather than their normal brown rice chicken-feed. Given whole rice once again, they recovered. In 1912, working at the Lister Institute in London, the Polish-born biochemist Casimir Funk isolated the active substances in rice husks which were preventing beriberi. He named such dietary missing links 'vitamines' (= 'vital amines') in the belief that they were amines, compounds derived from ammonia – the final 'e' in vitamins was dropped in 1920, when it became clear that not all vitamins were amines. Funk linked vitamin deficiency with such diseases as pellagra, beriberi but also scurvy and rickets. Deficiency syndromes had thus been identified in the laboratory, and the nutritional roles of various foods – vegetable products (leaves, stems, seeds), milk, egg yolk and meat – were in the process of being elucidated. A theoretical basis for nutrition had been established.

Study and action on undernutrition attained momentum between the First and Second World Wars. Economic depression in the West ('the hungry 1930s') and growing awareness of famine and starvation in the so-called Third World brought together laboratory scientists, clinicians and advocates of the importance of diet and 'lack' on health. Perhaps the most influential figure was John Boyd Orr (1880–1971), who spent his career fighting world hunger and undernutrition, working with organizations such as the United Nations to bring about worldwide changes in public health. A Scot, Boyd Orr founded the Rowett Research Institute in Aberdeen in 1922 and served as a director until 1945. He was also editor of the journal *Nutrition Abstracts and Reviews*, which drew attention to the universal problem of undernutrition. The UK only developed its first nutrition programme following Boyd Orr's 1936 report *Food, Health and Income*, which revealed an appalling amount of undernutrition, especially in the lower social groups. Boyd Orr statistically correlated poverty, poor nutrition and poor health. While presenting a frightening picture of undernutrition and suggesting that much was due to poverty, inequality and market forces, he recommended ways of reconciling the interests of agriculture and public health. Proposing a number of programmes for increasing world food production, he championed science as crucial to solving the problem of world hunger. Under his influence, the League of Nations established its Committee on Nutrition and he became the first director of the United Nations Food and Agriculture Organization. Boyd Orr received the Nobel Peace Prize for his work in 1949.

Over the last 50 years, poor countries have witnessed many changes in international thinking with regard to strategies for reducing undernutrition, driven by a variety of forces beyond their control. During the past half century, we have had the protein era, the energy gap, the food crisis, applied nutrition programmes, multisectoral nutrition planning, nutrition surveillance, food insecurity and livelihood strategies, and the micronutrient era, amongst others. Despite, but perhaps partly also because of these shifting technical strategies and 'fashions', they rarely reflected changes in the nature of nutritional problems on the ground in poor countries. Undernutrition remains a desperately neglected aspect of health sciences and services. The global community fails, despite abundant evidence about the importance of nutrition – and maternal and child nutrition in particular – to catalogue and act on the long-term effects of undernutrition on development and health. What is also desperately needed is the identification and application of proven interventions to reduce undernutrition, and to convince policy-makers to take national and international action.

The problem of undernutrition now

More than one-third – 3.5 million – of all child deaths annually, and 11 per cent of the total disease burden worldwide are estimated to be due to maternal and child undernutrition. Undernutrition encompasses stunting (defined by the anthropometric indicator low height-for-age, an index of faltering growth), wasting (commonly defined by low weight-for-height), and deficiencies of essential vitamins and minerals (collectively referred to as micronutrients). Being underweight, or low weight compared with that expected for a well-nourished child of that age and sex, can involve both wasting and/or stunting. In 2005, an estimated 20 per cent of children under 5 years of age in poor countries were regarded as underweight, with countries in South-Central Asia and eastern Africa having the highest proportions. As many as 40 countries were estimated to have a stunting prevalence of 40 per cent or more, including 23 in Africa and 16 in Asia (see Figure 9.1). Severe wasting had a global prevalence of 3.5 per cent or 19 million children, and is now erroneously referred to as Severe Acute Malnutrition or SAM; erroneously because chronic disease including HIV/AIDS and malabsorption cause as much wasting as does acute food insecurity.

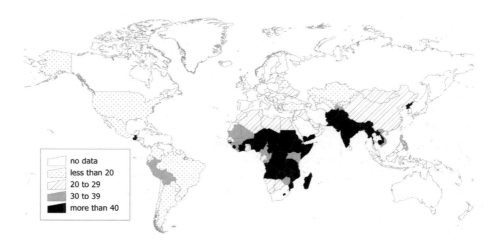

Figure 9.1 *Map showing the global distribution of prevalence of stunting in children under 5 years of age (%)*

Source: World Health Organization Statistical Information System at www.who.int/whosis (accessed on 17 February 2010)

The nutritional status of a woman before and during pregnancy is important for a healthy pregnancy and strong mother. Maternal undernutrition is associated with intrauterine growth restriction. Babies born at term (those who have completed 37 weeks of gestation), but of low birthweight (less than 2500 grams) are likely to have had intrauterine growth restriction. In poor countries it is estimated this is the case in 11 per cent of all live births. Maternal undernutrition has little effect on the volume or composition of breast milk unless undernutrition is severe. However, the concentration of some micronutrients (including vitamin A and iodine) in breast milk depends on the mother's nutritional status and intake. Iron deficiency anaemia is an underestimated indirect and important contributing factor to maternal mortality. Women of childbearing age are at high risk of iron deficiency anaemia because of blood loss during menstruation and the substantial iron demands of pregnancy.

A 2008 *Lancet* series on maternal and child malnutrition estimated that stunting, severe wasting and intrauterine growth restriction together were responsible for 2.2 million deaths of children under five years of age in 2005. Deficiencies in vitamin A and zinc had by far the highest disease burden in the micronutrients studied, and were estimated to be responsible for 600,000 and 400,000 million deaths, respectively. Iodine and iron deficiencies had smaller disease burdens, partly because of intervention programmes and the authors stressed the importance of a sustained effort. Sub-optimal breastfeeding was estimated to be responsible for 1.4 million child deaths.

Vitamin A deficiency is a common cause of preventable blindness. In addition, meta-analysis of randomized-controlled trials of vitamin A supplementation in young children in the early 1990s showed the importance of vitamin A in reducing the severity of infection and mortality. Vitamin A reduces the severity of diarrhoea and complications of measles, and the increased mortality from vitamin A deficiency is thought to be because of detrimental effects on the immune system.

Zinc is vital to protein synthesis, cellular growth and cellular differentiation. The health consequences of severe zinc deficiency have been elucidated over the past 40 years, whereas the health risks of mild to moderate deficiency have been described only recently. Clinical presentations of severe deficiency include growth retardation, impaired immune function, skin disorders, hypogonadism, anorexia and cognitive dysfunction. Mild to moderate deficiency increases susceptibility to infection, and the benefits of zinc supplementation on the immune system are well documented. Zinc deficiency in children results in increased risk of diarrhoea, pneumonia and malaria. Nowadays rehydration guidelines for children suffering from (acute or persistent) diarrhoea include a daily course of 20 milligrams of zinc.

Iodine is necessary for the thyroid hormones that regulate growth, development and metabolism and is essential to prevent goitre and cretinism. Inadequate intake can result in impairment of both intellectual development and physical growth.

Mainly found in haemoglobin, iron is essential for the binding and transportation of oxygen, as well as for the regulation of cell growth and differentiation. Iron deficiency is an important primary cause of anaemia, and chronic anaemia has detrimental effects on cognition. Other micronutrient deficiencies of concern include calcium, the B vitamins (especially folic acid and vitamin B12) and vitamin D.

Of great importance are the findings that indicators of undernutrition at age two years lead to large negative consequences in later life including shorter adult height, lower levels of schooling and reduced economic productivity, and for women, lower offspring birthweight. In addition, children who are undernourished in the first two years of life, and who put on weight rapidly later in childhood are at high risk of chronic non-communicable diseases related to nutrition, such as diabetes, hypertension and obesity (see also Chapter 10). Poorly nourished children may have delayed motor and cognitive development, which can lead parents to postpone the start of their children's schooling. These same children may progress through school more slowly, demonstrate poorer academic achievement, and perform less well on cognitive achievement tests when in school and later on during adulthood. Adults who were undernourished as children have been found to be less physically and intellectually productive. Cephalopelvic disproportion, implying disproportion between the head of the baby and the mother's pelvis, presenting a problem for safe childbirth, has been attributed to short stature in mothers resulting from stunting.

Nutrition and infection

> *Intensive research during the past 12 years on the relationship between diet and susceptibility to infection, not only in polio but also in common respiratory infections and tuberculosis, has convinced me that the human organism can protect itself against infection virtually completely by proper nutrition*
>
> Benjamin Sandler, 1951

There is a close but complex relationship between nutritional status and infectious disease. The social-medical historian Thomas McKeown argued in the 1960s and 1970s that improved nutrition accounted for most of the reduction in infectious diseases in Britain in the second half of the 19th century and early 20th century. His analyses for the period 1840–1950 show that by the time specific medical interventions such as vaccination and antibiotics were introduced in the 20th century, mortality from various infectious diseases had already declined by 80–90 per cent from their high rates in the mid-19th century. Mortality from tuberculosis, a disease closely associated with poverty, crowding and undernutrition, declined from around 4000 deaths per million per year in England and Wales in 1850 to around 400 per million by the time antibiotic treatment was introduced in the 1940s. The annual death rate from measles in children dropped from 1200 per million in the late 19th century to about one-tenth of that figure by the mid 1950s, when treatment of life-threatening secondary bacterial infections became possible. McKeown argued that gain in food production and overall wealth from the mid-19th century onwards in Britain improved the average levels of nutrition and that this increased resistance to infectious disease. Since the main declines were in diseases spread by inhalation such as tuberculosis, measles and diphtheria, McKeown reasoned that clean water was not a main benefactor. He concluded, therefore, that improved nutrition must have been important, shoring up bodily defences against all infections. More generally, his thesis drew attention to the profound influence of social and economic conditions as prime determinants of the health of populations.

Rehabilitation from childhood undernutrition: a continuum of care

While no one will argue that a sick child suffering from cerebral malaria or severe pneumonia needs to be treated in hospital immediately, there is still confusion on the optimal treatment in the clinical management and rehabilitation of severely undernourished children. The 1950s and 1960s were the period of hospital-based rehabilitation; in the 1970s the emphasis shifted to dedicated nutrition rehabilitation centres; the 1980s brought community- and home-based care of undernourished sick children. More recently, it is advocated that case management of children with undernutrition is best conducted within a District Health System based on the World Health Organization, UNICEF and partners' Integrated Management of Childhood Illnesses (IMCI) programme. This approach recognizes that nutrition rehabilitation does not take place in isolation and is a continuous process, a continuum between institution and community. Since the introduction of IMCI, simple and well-tested case management protocols for children with serious infections and/or severe undernutrition have become available.

These evidence-based protocols help to improve the case finding and management, and can reduce the unnecessarily high mortality rates in children with undernutrition admitted to health facilities. Hassan was treated according to IMCI guidelines at Bamyan hospital, discharged after 14 days and referred back to the community health worker for follow-up and inclusion in the village nutrition programme. This programme brings mothers together weekly for the preparation of a healthy and nourishing meal from the produce of a communal vegetable and fruit tree garden, as well as for health education and disease prevention sessions. When Hassan was seen by the mobile clinic team from the basic health centre in the catchment area one month later his weight had increased by 400 grams.

Undernutrition is not different from other health problems: prevention is clearly better than cure. Traditionally, programmes to improve the nutrition of children often begin by identifying undernourished children and then directing interventions at them. However, focusing on this might miss the crucial window of opportunity of providing for the high nutritional requirements from conception until the age of two, which are a pre-condition for 'producing' a healthy adult. The consequences of missing this window are irreversible, as the authors in *The Lancet* series on maternal and child undernutrition clearly show. Rather than only attempting to restore the nutritional status of children who are already undernourished, it is also of great importance to have interventions as well that prevent undernutrition in mothers during pregnancy and in young children during their first two years of life.

The diets of poor households in low-income countries often lack micronutrients and this is especially important for children. Dietary diversification, including the consumption of animal products or more fruits and vegetables, can help satisfy micronutrient requirements. Animal products are good sources of the most bio-available forms of vitamin A, iron and absorbable zinc, but they are also relatively high cost items. This is where the micronutrient food fortification with iodine and iron and/or supplementation programmes with vitamin A and zinc, as well as iron come in. These are highly cost-effective and proven interventions.

The World Health Organization and UNICEF recommend exclusive breastfeeding during the first six months of life. However, it is estimated that less than one-third of infants in poor countries receive this best practice. Improvement in breastfeeding (and weaning) practices is required, but needs realistic approaches in environments where women typically have to engage in agriculture and other labour intensive activities for many hours per day, and are frequently unable to keep their children with them. Implementation of the widely advocated education on the needs of pregnant and lactating women, of the importance of breastfeeding and on how to feed infants and young children (especially during episodes of illness), can have very beneficial impacts on the child's health and nutritional status. There is evidence that behavioural change can be a cost-effective way to improve nutrition. Households may not be able to afford to increase the amount of food they consume, but they may be able to change the way it is allocated among household members, or the type of food that is consumed, or the way it is prepared and served, in ways that can enhance nutrition. Delivering these messages effectively requires one-to-one discussion, typically with the mother. Breastfeeding promotion at the time of delivery in health facilities (in so-called 'baby-friendly' hospitals) can be highly cost-effective, but is only effective where a good proportion of deliveries occur in health facilities. Weighing the mother-to-be, and weighing and measuring the baby, are very important tools with which to frame the educational messages, as long as it is recognized that the weighing is not an end in itself – and this can be done outside the health facility in the community or household.

There seems to be a current bias in favour of programmes that address *micro*nutrient deficiencies relative to those that address the *macro*nutrients – the protein–energy deficiencies – and the tendency to view micronutrient deficiencies and protein–energy undernutrition as two separate problems. One wonders whether this is driven by the proven high cost-effectiveness of micronutrient interventions or whether this is determined by the technical nature and ease of implementation of these interventions relative to addressing overall undernutrition. Interventions that address undernutrition including protein–energy deficiencies are complicated to plan and implement, and require community and household participation in order to be successful – different from micronutrient interventions that can often be implemented 'top-down'.

Frustrated by years of developing recipes to help children recover from severe undernutrition that did not work, paediatric nutritionist André Briend was inspired by a jar of the chocolate spread Nutella. In 1996 he made his first cocktail of milk powder, sugar, peanut paste, oil, vitamins and minerals. His kitchen recipe has since been refined into a product commonly marketed as Plumpy'Nut. Plumpy'Nut and the concept of Ready to Use Therapeutic Food proved to be effective in the field (the first evidence came from Malawi and Ethiopia) and has now been endorsed by UNICEF, the World Health Organization and non-governmental organizations. What made Ready to Use Therapeutic Food revolutionary was that it provided the nutrients required to treat a severely undernourished child at home, without refrigeration, and even when hygiene conditions were not perfect. It is dispensed as foil-covered bars or in locally available plastic containers and can be stored in tropical conditions for three to four months. Most of the ingredients are available in many poor countries, but the milk powder, a main constitute of the paste, can be expensive.

Recent undernutrition health sector literature focuses on the interventions within the sector, such as micronutrient supplementation and food fortification programmes, hospital-based breastfeeding initiatives and limited community nutrition programmes. This might be partly related to the current dogma of having to show cost-effectiveness. There is a tendency in the cost-effectiveness literature to only consider interventions for which unit costs have been calculated and cost–benefit ratios have been worked out. Therefore, many worthwhile interventions are ignored, such as the provision of safe water or adequate sanitation, electricity and the expansion of female education, which have been shown to convincingly reduce child undernutrition but for which cost data have not been compiled and calculated. It is not clear how to use the cost-effectiveness framework to evaluate interventions in which nutritional improvement is only one of several objectives of these interventions. Unfortunately, too often such interventions, occurring outside the health sector, are lost in the discussion. However, in the medium to long term, interventions not directly related to the health sector such as improving agricultural productivity, infrastructure and logistics improvements, expanding female schooling, and fair trade agreements might have larger effects on the reduction of maternal and child undernutrition than nutritional supplementation or fortification programmes.

Effective nutrition action

The contemporary age is not short of terrible and nasty happenings, but the persistence of extensive hunger in a world of unprecedented prosperity is surely one of the worst.

Amartya Sen, 1999

Evidence about the many consequences of undernutrition for human, social and economic development constitutes a powerful reason for nutrition to move up the international, national and provincial or district scale. Yet, at all these levels the high prevalence of undernutrition in poor countries is not seen as anomalous, nor as a failure of those responsible to address the problem. Ignoring undernutrition rarely imposes political costs on leaders. Undernutrition, despite it being a key target ('between 1990 and 2015, halve the proportion of children under age five who are underweight') in relation to Millennium Development Goal One ('eradicate extreme hunger and poverty'), tends to be treated in policy processes as a business-as-usual issue. There is no drama associated with it; no perception that the issue is critical to the future of poor countries and poor people, the continued political success of governments, or the well-being of people. As a consequence, there is little political demand for action against undernutrition, and most governments of rich and poor countries do very little to ensure that nutrition-related goods and services are provided to poor people. Nutrition, which has few outspoken advocates, needs policy champions among senior officials in poor and rich countries.

A framework developed by UNICEF recognizes the basic and underlying causes of undernutrition, including the environmental, economic and socio-political contextual factors, with poverty having a central role (see Figure 9.2). This makes it explicit that multiple sectors need to be involved in any comprehensive effort to improve the nutritional status of populations, households and individuals. Undernutrition is not simply a medical problem that is solely addressed in a technical and scientific 'evidence-based' manner, but also a social problem of concern to many sectors. Another observation is that its underlying causes are related to one and another in complex ways. These interrelationships need to be analysed and properly understood in a given context to design appropriate remedies. For instance, food-secure households may still have undernourished children and women, because the burden of women's agricultural and other work or inadequate knowledge may compromise the quality of child care. Moreover, efforts to increase household food security may either increase or decrease levels of undernutrition depending on how these increases in production are achieved. And there are also situations in which culturally defined practices of food preparation or consumption may result in deficient or improper diets for young children or their mothers, which will need to be carefully addressed with community involvement.

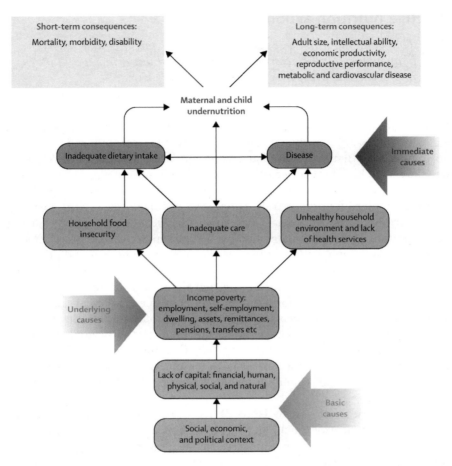

Figure 9.2 *Framework of the relations between poverty, food insecurity and other underlying and immediate causes to maternal and child undernutrition and its short-term and long-term consequences*

Source: Black, R.E. et al. *The Lancet* 2008; 371: 243–60

Undernutrition at the household level is clearly also affected by societal factors. That is, the availability of nutritional resources at the household level is linked to what happens at the macro-level. Over the past half-century global food production has increased dramatically and has outpaced population growth. These successes were achieved partly as the result of the use of new technologies including chemical fertilizers, pesticides and disease-resistant seeds. In addition, substantial additions to arable land have been made, also through widespread irrigation. Yet, despite this growth in food production a June 2009 World Food Programme report estimated a shocking record 1.02 billion people or almost one-sixth of the world's population as being undernourished. How is this possible? One reason is, as the economist

Amartya Sen has pointed out, that distribution of food supplies between and within countries is inequitable. He argues that many countries experiencing famine have adequate food supply for their populations; it is simply not distributed properly.

There is nothing new in this. During the catastrophic potato famine in Ireland in the mid-19th century, large quantities of cattle, corn and other foodstuffs were produced and exported to England in amounts that would have been quite adequate to avert the famine if the Irish people had had enough money to buy them. The British government reduced the price of grain in 1846 by repealing the Corn Laws in an effort to make grain more easily obtainable in Ireland. But the Irish tenant farmers grew grain in order to pay rent to their landowners: the falling price of grain simply increased their rent and hence their poverty. Of the estimated one million Irish deaths from the potato famine, many were directly due to starvation and many were due to outbreaks of infectious diseases. More recent famines in poor countries have shown similar chains of events. Inadequate distribution of food together with inadequate local production continues to beset many parts of the world. Some countries with borderline food production are in a particularly precarious situation because of the instability of world food prices and the variation in their own domestic production in different geographical areas of their countries, as well as wide differences in the purchasing power of individual households. Under these unstable conditions, famines may easily be precipitated by conflicts, floods and drought with crop failures due to unusual weather conditions (which might very well become increasingly not 'unusual' as they are related to climate change and global warming), and/or loss of purchasing power with high food prices.

Unfortunately, international food aid remains a major resource dominating nutritional interventions. The World Food Programme reported a total of US$2.7 billion in food aid and related resources in 2006, including about $1.5 billion to the 20 countries with the highest burden of undernutrition. Food aid continues to be used to support untargeted food distribution or school feeding programmes for which there is no proven effect on nutritional status. Another issue is that a disproportionate percentage of food aid goes to address acute food shortages as a result of crises. The plight of 2 million displaced people in Darfur in the Sudan is just one tragedy of the first decade of the new millennium. However, the vast majority, an estimated 90 per cent of the world's hungry people, are not victims of famine as a result of acute crises, but from chronic hunger – nagging 'quiet' hunger that does not go away. Additional funding is required that is applied in a comprehensive approach that addresses immediate, underlying and basic causes of undernutrition, and which requires more effective collaboration among all sectors that bear on maternal and child undernutrition. These include agriculture and rural development also using new technologies to improve the nutrient content of crops ('biofortication'), water and sanitation, and social development that takes account of health services, the education of girls and the empowerment of women. Other important sectors include financing, using innovative methods such as making available microfinance and conditional cash-transfer products to rural households, and trade (reform).

A panel of eight economic experts, including five Nobel laureates, was invited in 2008 by the Copenhagen Consensus Centre, a think-tank in Denmark, to set priorities among a series of 30 proposals for confronting 10 great global challenges: diseases, education, women and development, global warming, air pollution, conflicts, terrorism, subsidies and trade barriers, sanitation and water, and undernutrition and hunger. Ranking was done using cost-effectiveness analysis, but with the realization of its limitations and difficulties, as well as taking into account institutional preconditions for success and the demands of ethical and humanitarian urgency. Supplying the micronutrients vitamin A and zinc was ranked the highest priority by the expert panel, followed by trade reform. The third priority was fortifying foods with iron and iodized salt. The other seven of the top ten solutions included expanded immunization coverage of children, biofortification, de-worming, lowering the price of schooling, increasing girls' schooling, community-based nutrition promotion, and support for women's reproductive roles. My reservations about putting too much emphasis on cost-effectiveness analysis of individual solutions and 'either–or' solutions remain. However, these ten solutions plus others (water and sanitation interventions, and conditional cash-transfers were in the top 20) are important if we are to design comprehensive approaches to better address undernutrition.

The compelling logic of all this information is that governments need comprehensive national nutrition plans to scale-up relevant interventions, systems to monitor and evaluate those plans, and laws and policies to enhance the rights and status of women and children. Global leadership and negotiations that lead to new global treaties relevant to nutrition in trade, agriculture and poverty reduction are also needed. Coupled with more funding for nutrition from international donors, the result could be better targeted policies, with a shift away from the current domination of food aid and supply-led technical assistance to greater investment in human and institutional capacity building in poor countries. These reforms are long over-due.

Sources and suggestions for further reading

For the history of nutrition I made use of Roy Porter's *The Greatest Benefit to Mankind: A Medical History of Humanity* (London: W.W. Norton & Company, 1997), as well as Tony McMichael's *Human Frontiers, Environments and Disease* (Cambridge: Cambridge University Press, 2001). The classic, Thomas McKeown's *The Modern Rise of Population* (New York: Academic Press, 1976), can still be bought on-line, but for a price. The series of five papers on 'Maternal and Child Undernutrition' were published in *The Lancet* during January and February 2008. On the internet, www.who.int/child_adolescent_health/documents/malnutrition offers a set of very useful manuals with guidelines for the management of undernourished children. I made good use of the 2008 'challenge paper' on 'Hunger and malnutrition' by Sue Horton and others as well as the 'perspective paper' by Anil Deolalikar; both papers can be downloaded from the Copenhagen Consensus Centre website (www.copenhagenconsensus.com). This website also has the results of the Copenhagen Consensus 2008. Low- and middle-income countries that have improved nutritional status include Brazil, China, Costa Rica, Cuba, Sri Lanka and Thailand, and contributing factors to success are described in *Halving Hunger: It Can be Done* by the UN Millennium Project, Taskforce on hunger (London: Earthscan, 2005).

10
New diseases of poverty

It can be said that each civilization has a pattern of disease particular to it. The pattern of disease is an expression of the response of man to his total environment (physical, biological, and social); this response is, therefore, determined by anything that affects man or his environment.

René Dubos, 1961

Mariama

Mariama, around 35 five years young, lives in Banjul, the capital of The Gambia. And she does so comfortably: her husband is a high-ranking civil servant which enables her to employ two domestic staff who clean the house, cook and wash, and look after her four children. The chauffeur-driven government car, purchased with a loan from the World Bank, is available to help with the shopping, to bring the children to school, and to transport Mariama to visit her friends. At home and during these visits Mariama eats well, very well and sugar, salt, meat and oil are important ingredients of many dishes and snacks. Consequently, Mariama has the looks of a Rubens model, in agreement with the current local beauty ideal. Recently, Mariama did not feel well, and her husband arranged an urgent appointment with one of the few internal medicine specialists in (part-time) government service in the country. This doctor diagnosed hypertension and obesity, and Mariama also had an impaired glucose tolerance test. Medication was prescribed for one month and Mariama was given a new appointment. Unfortunately she was not given any advice on diet or exercise. The cost of the first consultation was four times The Gambia's per capita health budget per year.

Mariama is not the only one suffering from so-called diseases of affluence. In a study we did during the late 1990s more than 30 per cent of the Banjul women aged 35–54 were obese. In addition, almost 20 per cent of all adults participating in this survey had high blood pressure, and 8 per cent had diabetes mellitus. A similar prevalence survey in a rural population showed significantly lower levels of hypertension, and almost no diabetes mellitus or overweight according to international guidelines. At the same time, there was still much undernutrition, almost 20 per cent of men and women, rural and urban, young and not so young adults.

Diet and disease

In rural Africa, and much of South Asia, over half of the dietary energy comes from cereals or less often, starchy roots or fruits. By contrast, in Europe and North America, less than a quarter of total energy comes from cereals. With the industrial and technological revolution that began around 200 years ago in Britain and subsequently spread through Europe, North America and eventually other countries and regions, we have developed technologies for food production, processing and storage. These provide populations with a year-round supply of foods that have artificially high concentrations of energy, fat and sugar. The level of consumption of added fats, dairy products, salt, sweeteners and alcohol in 'Western diets' is generally inversely related to the consumption of starchy staples.

The Irish surgeon Dennis Burkitt, with long experience in East Africa, observed in the 1970s that a number of diseases such as cardio-vascular disease (including stroke), diabetes mellitus, obesity, dental decay, appendicitis, diverticulitis, gallstone disease, large bowel cancer, haemorrhoids and varicose veins were extremely uncommon in the traditional rural populations in the region. He postulated that in the development of these diseases, that were so common in rich countries, changes in the diet were playing an important role.

At the beginning of the 20th century, cardiovascular disease was responsible for less than 10 per cent of all deaths worldwide, but by the beginning of the 21st century that figure had risen to 30 per cent. By 2001, cardiovascular disease had become the leading cause of death in the so-called developing world, as it had been in many rich countries since the mid 1900s. Over the past two centuries, the industrial and technological revolutions have resulted in a dramatic shift in the causes of illness and death. Before 1900, infectious diseases and undernutrition were the most common causes of death worldwide; however after 1900 they were gradually replaced in most rich countries by cardiovascular disease and cancer.

High blood pressure or hypertension became the high-profile heart condition of the 20th century, being a major risk factor for heart attacks. Arteriosclerosis – thickening and hardening of the arteries – means that the heart must beat more strongly to perfuse the body with blood; this produces the 'hard pulse' familiar to clinicians, strains the heart and brings shortness of breath and angina chest pains. Atherosclerosis, a form of arteriosclerosis that is caused by a build up of fatty deposits in arterial walls, is also associated with stress, smoking and excessive drinking. A sudden occlusion of a coronary artery causes a heart attack, sometimes with loss of heart rhythm which may prove fatal. Cardiac catheterization was developed in the 1930s, leading to modern angiocardiography. This was later augmented by the development of non-invasive methods of studying the heart such as computerized axial tomography (CAT)-scanning and nuclear magnetic resonance (NMR)-imaging. Diagnostic advance was also accompanied by progress in managing hypertensive heart disease; coronary artery bypass and other open heart surgery to relieve the occluded arteries that caused angina and heart attacks was introduced from the 1960s. Drug treatments for failing hearts were steadily improved. What also contributed to falling coronary heart disease in a number of rich countries were the moves to healthier lifestyles. This occurred from the 1970s onwards, consequent upon better understanding of preventing the causes of much heart disease. The breakthrough came through chemistry.

The dangers of atherosclerosis, or the laying of fatty plaques in the walls of arteries, had become clear. The main component of such arterial plaques was found by the Americans Michael Brown and Joseph Goldstein to be cholesterol, manufactured in the liver and supplemented by fat-rich foodstuffs. In 1985 they were the co-receivers of the Nobel Prize for Medicine 'for their discoveries concerning the regulation of the cholesterol mechanism'. This reinforced the findings of epidemiologists and medical statisticians that the affluent were more prone to heart disease than the poor: rich people had richer diets. Understanding the role of cholesterol promoted new ideas about diet and drugs in the prevention of heart attacks and strokes caused by the clogging of arteries. Public understanding of risk factors – smoking, diet, obesity, lack of exercise – improved, and lifestyle shifts made a fundamental contribution to reducing the problem. Sales of butter and other dairy products dropped in many rich countries while purchases of vegetable oils containing polyunsaturated fats rose, adding salt to food was reduced and jogging became fashionable. Partly as a consequence coronary heart disease in the US dropped by half between 1970 and 1990 – a reduction of 300,000 deaths a year – and there was also a substantial decline in strokes. However, improvement was not uniform and there has been a shift in the burden from rich to poor in Western countries. In Britain, in the early 1970s the rate of early death from coronary heart disease was 1.2 times larger in the lowest social class than in the highest social class. By the early 1990s the ratio had increased to around 2.2. As shown in Figure 10.1, cardiovascular disease deaths are now also higher in many low- and middle-income countries compared to high-income countries.

This shift from the rich to the poor might be partly explained by the 'foetal origins' theory. In the 1990s, the Englishman David Barker hypothesized, supported by epidemiological and animal experimental evidence, that experiences of foetal life, especially when there is suboptimal maternal nutrition, 'programme' foetal growth and metabolism in ways that enhance immediate survival, but which may compromise good health in adult life. There is reasonably good evidence that the adult risks of several major diseases, including heart disease, stroke and diabetes, are increased in low

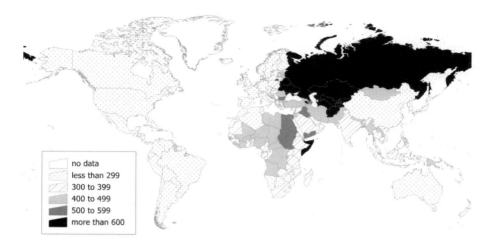

Figure 10.1 *Map showing the global distribution of cardiovascular disease death rates (age-standardized mortality rate per 100,000 population)*

Source: World Health Organization Statistical Information System at www.who.int/whosis (last accessed on 17 February 2010)

birthweight babies or, in some studies, in babies with thin bodies. These two types of growth deficit reflect undernutrition at different stages of foetal life, and affect, respectively, blood pressure and insulin action. Barker argues that this leads to increased susceptibility to adult cardiovascular disease and diabetes, and that this occurs when a growth-retarded foetus and low birthweight baby, 'programmed' to survive on 'lean fuel' becomes an overweight individual in well-fed adult life. This might very well be what happened to Mariama, and with her to many other men and women in poor countries where low birth weight is more common than in rich countries, and more so in lower social classes in most studies.

Big tobacco

The boys visiting the local discotheque of Farafenni on this Saturday evening in 1999, a border place 200km upcountry from Banjul, are being presented with free cigarettes that are also being lit for them by attractive young women in Marlboro uniform. I have seen this before, but cannot stop becoming upset and angry once again. I look for the manager of this 'marketing-campaign' who is standing outside the discotheque next to a new SUV car, covered, of course, with large Marlboro signs. I try to convey my message that he will bear responsibility for the cigarette addiction of these disco-boys, and in the long term for the death of many of them. He and the bystanders look at me uncomprehendingly and laugh at me. I go home even more upset and angry.

The Gambian government cancelled a ban on cigarette advertising in 1998, and a reason for this was not given. However, it had been the Minister of Finance who managed to convince his colleagues of the necessity of this measure. Whether there were other 'arguments' which made it difficult for the Ministers to say no to the proposal of their finance colleague, we will probably never know. The protests by the Gambian Medical Association were not listened to.

The link between the smoking of cigarettes and lung cancer began to be suspected by clinicians in Germany and elsewhere in the 1930s when they noted an increase in this 'unusual' disease. The suspicion was based on the fact that many patients who acquired lung cancer were also smokers. Although this was an astute observation, these workers lacked the scientific evidence to justify their position. As a result, between 1930 and 1960, numerous epidemiological studies were undertaken to try to quantify the relationship between cigarette smoking and lung cancer. Two of these studies, by Sir Richard Doll and Austin Bradford Hill, are considered classics. Doll and Hill first used the case-control study method and compared the smoking history of a large sample of hospital patients with lung cancer with the smoking history of a similar group without lung cancer. This study, published in 1950 concluded that 'The risk of developing the disease increases in proportion to the amount smoked. It may be fifty times as great among those who smoke twenty-five or more cigarettes a day as among non-smokers'. Doll himself stopped smoking as a result of these findings. In 1954, the first results of a cohort study by Doll and Hill of the smoking habits of 40,000 medical practitioners were published, which confirmed the results of the earlier study. In 1964 the US Surgeon-General found that death from cancer overall among men who smoked was 70 per cent higher than for non-smokers. Then in a 1979 report the Surgeon General announced that, above the increased risk of cancer the biggest risk from smoking was heart disease. Despite good evidence of this relationship having been 'discovered' more than 50 years ago, now more people than ever – 1.1. billion – smoke cigarettes. How did this happen?

I think this is mainly because it is profitable to producers, tobacco company shareholders and governments. In addition the product is recognized as highly addictive. Smoking is increasing in many of the poorer parts of the world. An estimated 930 million of the 1.1 billion smokers live in the so-called developing world. For an overview of the percentage of adults who smoke cigarettes per country see Figure 10.2. Tobacco, which is estimated to kill half of the people who use it, is increasingly a leading cause of health inequalities between poor and rich populations. Much of the global increase is the result of the hard selling campaigns by rich multinationals, which have shifted their attention to new markets with less regulation – the poor countries. The tobacco industry continues to spend tens of billions of dollars each year on marketing, including traditional advertising (e.g. broadcast and print advertisements, billboards), point-of-sale materials in stores, indirect marketing (e.g. sponsoring of sporting and cultural events, charitable

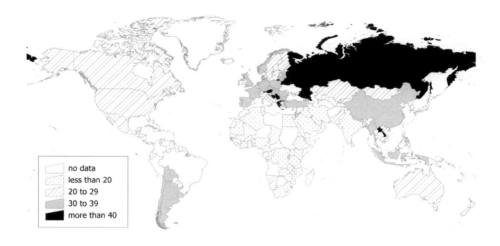

Figure 10.2 *Map showing the global distribution of smoking among adults (%)*

Source: World Health Organization Statistical Information System at www.who.int/whosis (accessed on 17 February 2010)

contributions, promotional allowances to wholesalers, distributors and retailers, free cigarettes, in-store product displays and branded promotional items), public relations and lobbying including politicians, and targeted price discounts to offset taxation. Smoking is also still frequently portrayed in movies, often placed, supported and paid for by the tobacco industry despite prohibitions on such practices in many countries.

The epidemiological transition

If children were still dying at 1978 rates, there would have been 16.2 million deaths globally in 2007. In fact, there were 'only' 9.2 million such deaths. This difference of 7.0 million deaths is not only equivalent to more than 18,000 children's lives being saved every day, it also 'lengthens' life expectancy. As the burden of infectious diseases that have their highest toll amongst young children declines, the demographic transition that was discussed (see Chapter 5) will lead to an epidemiological transition: an age-related shift in the profile of diseases. The so-called diseases of affluence or lifestyle that are often equated with chronic non-communicable diseases – mainly cardiovascular disease, obesity, cancer, chronic respiratory diseases and diabetes thus become more common in longer-living populations. Because gains in life expectancy occurred first in the richer section of rich countries, cardiovascular disease and other chronic non-communicable diseases emerged early on in that section. However, as behaviours such as cigarette smoking and eating high-fat, high-sugar and salt rich diets became mass phenomena, and eventually more prevalent among the poorer sections, so the socio-economic distribution of most of these diseases reversed. The adverse health impacts of socio-economic disadvantage and associated chronic life stress increased the relationship between individual poverty and health.

Recently, poorer countries have incurred what is being called a 'double burden of disease'. One burden arises from the fact that economic progress as well as establishing modern public health and medical care has bypassed the bottom billion who continue to suffer heavily from infectious diseases, maternal and perinatal conditions and undernutrition. Meanwhile, the other burden in these poorer countries is the rise in chronic non-communicable disease as a consequence of population ageing, urbanization and altered consumer behaviours. Cardiovascular disease, obesity, cancers, chronic respiratory disease, diabetes but also mental health problems and injuries (especially on the roads) are becoming the leading causes of disability and premature death in most regions of the world.

Chronic non-communicable diseases were estimated to cause more than 60 per cent (35 million) of global deaths in 2005; more than 80 per cent of these deaths occurred in poorer countries. The low priority that is given to chronic non-communicable diseases at a global level is surprising because they are a major impediment to human development. Chronic non-communicable diseases impose large health and economic burdens on poor countries. Poverty is an important cause of chronic non-communicable diseases and these diseases contribute to poverty, especially where out-of-pocket payments for health care are the norm. The under appreciation of chronic non-communicable diseases as development issues as well as the underestimation of their economic effects has resulted in many governments as well as the global health community taking too little interest in their prevention and leaving this responsibility primarily to individuals. This indifference is unjustified. The World Health Organization has proposed a global goal for the prevention and control of chronic diseases to complement the Millennium Development Goals. This goal is for an additional 2 per cent reduction per year of deaths attributable to these diseases, and achievement of the global goal would avert an estimated 36 million deaths by 2015. Estimates have shown that over 70 per cent of cardiovascular disease deaths, around 40 per cent of chronic respiratory disease deaths, 34 per cent of cancer deaths and about 50 per cent of all chronic disease deaths are attributable to a small number of known modifiable risk factors. In addition, because many of these averted deaths would be in poor countries and half would be in people younger than 70 years, it would have major economic benefits, including an extension of productive life and a reduction in the need for expensive care. Is this goal achievable?

Prevention and management of the so-called diseases of affluence

Modern medicine has developed the capacity, through late stage crisis management and at enormous cost, to add a few extra months or years of life for smokers who would otherwise have died of coronary heart failure or lung cancer. The blessing to the lucky individual may be inestimable, but that hardly counts in the global health statistics. The contribution of prolonging some coronary insufficiency associated heart failure or lung cancer patients' lives is rather slight: most who have been diagnosed and treated with these conditions do not live more than five years. Estimations by health economists suggest that the money spent on these forms of cardiology and oncology would be more wisely spent on prevention and early treatment of risk factors.

To prevent death or illness from chronic non-communicable diseases in a sustainable manner, an intervention should meet at least four conditions. First, the intervention must target most risk factors that have been causally associated with chronic non-communicable diseases. Second, there should be knowledge that the intervention will probably lead to favourable changes in the risk factors, which should then lead to reductions in disease and death. Third, evidence should – where possible – show that the intervention is cost-effective in the settings in which it is implemented. Lastly, there should be evidence that a scaling up of the intervention is financially feasible in poor countries.

In terms of their effectiveness, cost, acceptability, and feasibility, salt reduction and tobacco control are two population-based strategies high on the priority list for global implementation. There is good evidence that a moderate reduction of salt intake to less than the recommended 5 grams per day can be achieved by a voluntary reduction of the salt content of processed foods by manufacturers, plus a sustained campaign aimed to encourage dietary change within households and communities with the message 'avoid salty food' and 'do not add salt at the table'. This can reduce the blood pressure by a small but important amount, with a greater decrease in blood pressure in people with higher baseline blood pressures. The 2005 World Health Organization Framework Convention on Tobacco Control proposed a set of policies to reduce demand for tobacco. These include increased taxes on tobacco products, enforcement of smoke-free public- and work-places, requirements for packaging and labelling of tobacco products combined with public awareness campaigns about the health risks, and a comprehensive ban on smoking advertising, promotion and sponsorship. A 2007 series on chronic diseases in *The Lancet* estimated that over 10 years (2006–2015) the deaths of almost 14 million people, from 23 low- and middle-income countries for which estimates were done, could be averted if these selected measures to reduce tobacco and salt exposure were implemented. Total expenditure for implementation of both strategies was estimated at between US$0.14 and $0.38 per person per year for poorer countries; most of the cost would be spent on legislation measures, and enforcement of these as well as awareness campaigns.

Other population-based strategies with good potential but insufficient evidence include 'cooking oils control' and weight reduction via increased physical activity in addition to dietary advice. A government led programme in Mauritius that changed the cooking oils from a predominantly saturated-fat palm oil to soybean oil high in unsaturated fats led to a significant reduction in cholesterol concentrations. More evidence is needed from different settings, but such a 'cooking oils control' strategy has potentially large benefits.

Modest weight loss – 5–10 per cent – in those with excess weight is associated with a significant improvement in blood pressure in individuals with and without hypertension, as well as improvements in cholesterol and glucose tolerance. There is insufficient consensus on the single dietary approach to weight reduction, but there is agreement that those that include physical activity in addition to dietary advice are more successful. And although there are no large-scale randomized controlled trials (the gold-standard for showing that an intervention is efficacious), a large number of studies show clear evidence of a relationship between increased physical activity and lower all-cause mortality in men and women of all ages.

Unlike high-technology approaches, a simple multi-drug regimen of aspirin, blood pressure-lowering drugs and cholesterol-lowering drugs, with health promotion advice for individuals at high risk of cardiovascular disease, could relatively easily be brought to scale in poor countries, since it could be delivered mainly through primary health care and outpatient settings. Most people at high risk can be easily identified by their personal or family history of a heart attack, stroke or other major cardiovascular event. Others can be identified with easily measurable risk factors (including history of alcohol and tobacco use, age, sex, blood pressure, body mass index) that do not require expensive and time-consuming laboratory testing. This approach to scaling up a multi-drug regimen plus health education for individuals with existing cardiovascular disease or who are at high risk of cardiovascular disease could avert almost 18 million deaths from the 23 low- and middle-income countries analysed in *The Lancet* chronic diseases series, at a cost of less than $1 per person per year in poor countries, or $55 per treated individual per year. This cost includes resources spent on medicines, health service delivery for screening and treatment, laboratory testing and programme costs related to administration, training, monitoring and assessment of the programme.

Another individual-based strategy is the prevention of progression to diabetes from impaired glucose tolerance by lifestyle interventions focusing on a healthy diet and increasing physical activity, if necessary in combination with cheap oral drugs. Studies in China and India have shown that such interventions can reduce the progression to diabetes mellitus. The blood-glucose testing needed to detect glucose intolerance, as well as the successful management of diabetes and other chronic diseases or risk factors such as hypertension can be done very well by nurses in primary care settings. However, in this case also, more evidence of the cost-effectiveness and sustainability of such approaches in other countries is urgently needed.

Mariama was lucky; one of her friends had similar health problems. The friend had received advice from her doctor on a healthy diet and regular physical exercise. They 'joined forces', by making changes in their diet and by going to the gym together. Mariama was able to reduce her weight, her blood pressure came down and repeat glucose tolerance tests became normal. After six months she was off medication, and perhaps more important – she felt much better and fitter.

If nothing is done to reduce the risk of chronic non-communicable diseases, an estimated $84 billion of economic production will be lost because of heart disease, stroke and diabetes alone in the 23 low- and middle-income countries analysed in *The Lancet* chronic diseases series between 2006 and 2015. Achievement of the global goal for chronic non-communicable diseases prevention and control – an additional 2 per cent annual reduction in chronic non-communicable disease death rates over this period – would avert 24 million deaths in these countries, and would save an estimated $8 billion, which is almost 10 per cent of the projected loss in national income due to these diseases during the 10 year period. Almost 80 per cent of the years of life gained would be from deaths averted in people younger than 70 years, and 57 per cent from deaths averted in those younger than 60 years.

Early childhood development

Each one of you is your own person, endowed with rights, worthy of respect and dignity. Each one of you deserves to have the best possible start in life, to complete a basic education of the highest quality, to be allowed to develop your full potential and provided the opportunities for meaningful participation in your communities.

Nelson Mandela and Graça Machel, 2000

The vast majority of the more than 9 million children who die each year before their fifth birthday worldwide, are born in low- or middle-income countries, and within these countries, are children of more disadvantaged households and communities. There is an urgent need to address these mortality inequities. Less obvious but equally important are the 200 million children who are not achieving their full development potential. Experiences in early childhood lay critical foundations for the entire life-course. For the individual child and for society it is better to provide a positive start rather than to resort to remedial action later on. Building on the well recognized and successful safe motherhood and child survival agendas, governments and civil society organizations can make major and sustained improvements in population health and development by adopting a more comprehensive approach to ensuring a healthy early life, starting in pre-pregnancy and continuing through pregnancy and childbirth, to the early days and years of life.

As previously described, good evidence suggests that the risks among adults of several chronic non-communicable diseases, including heart disease, stroke and diabetes, is increased in low birthweight babies. Equally important, the science of early childhood development shows that brain development is highly sensitive to external influences in early childhood. This starts in utero and has lifelong effects. The conditions to which children are exposed, including the quality of their relationships and their language environment, literally 'sculpt' the developing brain. Raising healthy children means stimulating their physical, language/cognitive and social/emotional development. Healthy development during the early years provides essential building blocks that enable individuals to flourish in many domains, including social, emotional, cognitive and physical well-being.

Education, preschool and beyond, fundamentally shapes children's lifelong trajectories and opportunities for health. Yet despite recent progress, there are an estimated 75 million children of primary school age who are not in school. Educational attainment is linked to improved health outcomes, partly through the effect of health on adult income, employment and living conditions. There are also strong intergenerational effects. The educational attainment of mothers is a determinant of child health, child survival and child educational attainment. Many health challenges in adult life have their roots in the early years of life, including cardiovascular disease, diabetes and obesity. Social inequalities contribute to inequities in health later on. Children from disadvantaged backgrounds are more likely to do poorly in school and, as adults, are more likely to have low incomes and high fertility rates, and be less empowered to seek good health care, and/or to provide good nutrition and stimulation to their own children, thus contributing to the intergenerational transmission of disadvantage.

The health care system plays a pivotal role in early child survival and development. Mothers and children need a continuum of care from pre-pregnancy, through pregnancy and childbirth, to the early days and years of life. They need safe and healthy environments including good quality housing, clean water and adequate sanitation facilities, safe neighbourhoods and protection against violence. Good nutrition is crucial and begins in utero with adequately nourished mothers, underlining the importance of taking a life-course perspective in tackling health inequalities. It is important to support the initiation of early breastfeeding and exclusive breastfeeding in the first six months of life; this is as important as ensuring the availability of and access to healthy diets for infants and young children through improving food security.

Early child survival and development depend on how well and how equitably societies, governments and international organizations organize their affairs. Gender equity, through maternal education, income-generating opportunities and empowerment play an important role in child survival and development. Children benefit when national governments adopt family-friendly social protection policies. Children need support, nurturing, care and responsive living environments. And they need opportunities to explore their world, to play, to learn how to speak and listen to others. Schools are part of the environment that contributes to children's development, and have a vital role to play in building children's capabilities and, if they are truly inclusive, in achieving health equity.

Investments in early childhood development are some of the most powerful actions that societies can make in terms of both reducing the burden of chronic non-communicable diseases in adults, and in enabling more children to grow into healthy adults who can make a positive contribution to society, socially and economically. Investment in early childhood development can also be an important 'equalizer', since these interventions have the largest effects on the most deprived children.

While the benefits of early childhood development programmes are increasingly being recognized, there is also inadequate investment in this area. Studies by the World Bank and other agencies in low- and middle-income countries have shown benefit to cost ratios on early childhood development programming of around 3:1, meaning that for each dollar spent, there are three dollars of savings to society. These returns increase in programmes that target children most at risk. The conclusion is clear. As the World Bank economists Van der Gaag and Tan stated, 'Societies cannot prosper if their children suffer. Early childhood development programmes are a sound investment in the well-being of children and the future of societies. By breaking the intergenerational cycle of deprivation, early childhood development programmes are a powerful tool for obtaining the ultimate objective of development by giving people a chance to live productive and fulfilling lives.'

While arguing that we should invest in early childhood development programmes, I do not mean to imply that the living conditions of adults should not be corrected by persuading individuals to change their lifestyles or by treating and caring for people with chronic non-communicable diseases. What I am saying is that we need to do both.

Sources and suggestions for further reading

Roy Porter's *The Greatest Benefit to Mankind: A Medical History of Humanity* (London: W.W. Norton & Company, 1997), has been my main source of information on the history of the so-called diseases of affluence. It remains a magnificently readable and at the same time encyclopaedic book. For an excellent account of human health over time, and our interaction with the environment, including diet, please read Tony McMichael's publication *Human Frontiers, Environment and Disease* (Cambridge: Cambridge University Press, 2001). David Barker's *Mothers, Babies and Diseases in Later Life* (London: BMJ Publishing Group, 1994) is an account of the studies by Barker and his colleagues, which show that the nutrition of the foetus and newborn infant has significant effects on the health of the adult. The 'classics' by Doll and Hill can be found under R. Doll, A. Bradford Hill 'Smoking and carcinoma of the lung: Preliminary report' (*British Medical Journal* 1950; 2: 739–748, reprinted in 1999 in the *Bulletin of the World Health Organization*, 77: 84–93) and R. Doll and A. Bradford Hill, 'The mortality of doctors in relation to their smoking habits: A preliminary report', *British Medical Journal* (1954; ii: 1451–1455, reprinted in 2004 in the *British Medical Journal*, 328: 1529–1533). The chronic diseases series in *The Lancet* was published in 2007 between 8 December and 22/29 December. A good introduction to the subject of early childhood development can be found in *From Early Childhood Development to Human Development* (edited by Mary Eming Young, published by The World Bank, Washington, DC, 2002), which addresses the benefits and challenges of investing in early childhood development. The results of rural–urban comparison in The Gambia of chronic non-communicable diseases risk factors are reported in Marianne van der Sande et al. 'Blood pressure patterns and cardiovascular risk factors in rural and urban Gambian communities', *Journal of Human Hypertension (*2000; 14: 489–496) and 'Obesity and undernutrition and cardiovascular risk factors in rural and urban Gambian communities', *American Journal of Public Health* (2001; 91: 1641–1644). Salt reduction, resulting in lower blood pressure levels, was achieved in community-based trials in China, Jamaica and Nigeria (H. Tian et al. *Journal of Human Hypertension* 1995; 9: 959–968, and T. Forrester et al., *Journal of Human Hypertension* (2005; 19: 55–60). The Tianjin project in China showed reductions in hypertension and obesity (Yu Z et al. *Preventative Medicine* 1999; 29: 165–172). The community-based Mauritius project included a government-led programme that changed the main cooking oil from a predominantly saturated-fat palm oil to a soybean oil high in unsaturated fatty acids, resulting in lower overall cholesterol concentrations (U. Uusitalo et al. *British Medical Journal* 1996; 313: 1044–1046). Prevention of a progression to diabetes from impaired glucose tolerance with lifestyle interventions has been demonstrated in China (G. Li et al. *Lancet* 2008; 371: 1783–1789), while nurse-led management for diabetes and hypertension in rural South Africa resulted in successful control of the disorders in a high proportion of patients (R. Coleman et al. *Bulletin of the World Health Organization* 1998; 76: 633–640).

11
Health financing

Anyone who has ever struggled with poverty knows how extremely expensive it is to be poor.

James Baldwin, 1961

Helena

It is a very warm afternoon, and I am glad that I am being asked to sit on a stool in the shadow of the hut. After the usual elaborate greetings, Helena tells me in the local language, translated to me in Kiswahili by the local community leader, that her husband is not around. He left her six months ago. I continue with my questionnaire. Helena has never attended school, has no radio or bicycle, no livestock and no corrugated roof on her hut which has two small rooms where she and her five children live, sleep, eat and cook. At the same time, the compound is clean, there is a separate area for waste disposal, a good pit latrine, and three clay pots out of the sun filled with drinking water. The larger children go to school, the younger ones have 'road to health' cards showing regular attendance at the clinic for growth monitoring and full vaccination coverage.

I explain to Helena that the Tanzanian government has introduced 'cost sharing' in the national health system. And that I am part of a team that is doing a survey on willingness and ability to pay to see what is feasible in our district. At the same moment I realize that I can answer the questions that are to follow. One can't ask Helena to contribute, this single mother-cum-subsistence farmer has nothing, absolutely nothing. Cost-sharing is not as simple as it is thought to be in New York, Washington, London and Dar es Salaam. Helena indicates that she, as nine others out of ten interviewed, prefers a community-based health financing scheme above user fees. On the question how much she will be able to contribute, she thinks carefully before answering and mentions an amount that seems realistic to her. The amount won't even match the administration costs of registering her in the scheme.

Health expenditure

During the 1980s, the cost, and therefore the financing of health care moved high on the agenda of health policy discussions. The subject was discussed at the Executive Board of the World Health Organization in 1986, and subsequently at the World Health Assembly in 1987. The concern applied to both rich and poor countries. The rich countries were concerned to find ways to contain the costs, while the poor countries were concerned to maintain and, if possible, increase expenditure, to implement policies that could achieve 'health for all'. Before the 1980s, many poor countries were restricted in what they could spend on health care due to the extremely limited supply of health professionals. They did not have enough doctors, nurses and allied health professionals to expand their health services. Since then, training programmes have produced a good increase in health professionals, albeit still insufficient in many poor countries. More recently the situation has become more difficult in many poor countries with the exodus and 'brain-drain' of qualified health workers to rich countries regarded by them as greener pastures.

But still, in the 1980s the increase in the human resource 'supply' as well as an increase in the number of facilities, including hospitals, which in considerable numbers were built and equipped from donations and loans, led to a pressure to increase public health expenditure especially for operating costs. The availability of new services and easier access increased demand, as more people sought help from 'modern' medical services rather than, or in addition to, traditional services. Some of this demand was also promoted by the health services and systems themselves as they encouraged children to come for immunization, pregnant women for antenatal, delivery and postpartum care, and patients with chronic cough to check their sputum for tuberculosis.

Other factors were (and are) the demographic and epidemiological transitions that have resulted in population increases including an increase in the number of older people who are larger users of health services and the double burden of infectious and chronic non-communicable diseases. And there is the factor of the development of new technologies. While the price of old drugs tends to fall, the price of new drugs is often very high indeed. And a vast range of new equipment has been developed to assist in the task of diagnosis and treatment. Often this does not replace older equipment, which is still needed, but is an extra supplement to what was there already. This new equipment needs further staff and materials to operate and maintain it. In addition to all of this, the world plunged into a severe economic recession during the 1980s.

The economic crisis

The initial cause of the economic crisis was the sharp increase in oil prices in 1982, initiated by OPEC, the cartel of oil-producing countries. The low- and middle-income countries which were not oil producers were immediately faced with what is now called a credit-crunch. Their exports were not sufficient to finance the import of oil at much higher prices, in addition to other needs. Many high-income countries reduced other imports so that the necessary oil could be bought at the higher prices. This had a further effect on the balance of payments of poor countries as the world demand for and therefore the prices of their raw materials declined sharply. Consequently, poor countries had to export more to earn the same amount of foreign exchange. When they were unable to do this, they were forced to devalue their currencies and seek loans from the International Monetary Fund, which in turn laid down terms which required a closer balance between tax revenue and public expenditure. This could most readily be achieved by cutting the latter. And the areas of public expenditure which were most often cut were the social sectors – mainly health and education, while the vast spending on defence often remained intact. In the health sector the cuts were often greater in (rural) primary health care, rather than (urban) secondary or tertiary care. The results of the so-called 'structural adjustment programmes' had devastating effects on poor people in poor countries. The real benefits of structural adjustment were enjoyed by the rich world with cheaper coffee, cotton, cocoa and so on.

Meanwhile the oil producers were placing their large profits in the leading banks in rich countries. These banks in turn searched for profitable and safe investments for the funds they were holding. The poor countries became the targets for lending on an enormous scale. It was believed that investments guaranteed by governments were bound to be safe. Often these funds were not put to use in strengthening local economies but in postponing politically unpopular measures which would increase tax revenues or decrease public expenditure. Moreover some funds returned to the banks in the rich countries as secret deposits of the politicians and high ranking civil servants handling the loans. Thus the strains on the balance of payments caused by the higher oil prices were followed by even greater strains in trying to pay the service charges due to foreign debts. And with devaluations these debt service payments became even larger in terms of the local currency.

Overall, the economic crisis resulted in declining public health financing. Ministries of Health typically responded with postponement of the maintenance of buildings, non-replacement of equipment and vehicles, and the undersupplying of drugs, other medical products and petrol. At the same time staff salaries were allowed to fall in real terms. Ministries of Health did not substantially cut staff, although those who often left were not replaced. Owing to the absence of vehicles and petrol, staff in outpost health facilities were no longer supervised. Patient numbers started falling when the supply of drugs and other essentials became uncertain. Staff responded to the lack of demand and the fall in their pay by spending less time at their jobs. Instead they engaged in other activities to support themselves and their families, including demanding illicit payments from patients for their services. The reaction of a large number of poor countries, including Tanzania, on this breakdown of the government health system, was to look for additional sources of finance for their health services. As foreign aid for health stagnated during the 1980s, poor countries had to look for additional resources from inside the country. One obvious source of revenue was to introduce or increase user fees for public health services, and Tanzania introduced these in a phased manner from 1993.

User fees

> *I think it is very important to have the patients, the people who ask for health services to pay. How that payment will be made ... it can be in a variety of ways. But the important thing is they must pay. They must feel it is a service they are buying, so that they feel equal, so that they don't feel small.*
>
> Muhammad Yunus, 2007

Few health policy issues are as controversial as user fees for health care. The case for charging individual patients for health services has been argued as preventing unnecessary or 'frivolous' use of health services, that patients are paying considerable amounts to private health providers including traditional healers and that therefore similar charges could be made for public health services, that patients should pay at least the marginal cost of what is provided, and that charges will enable services to be improved.

The argument that patients make unnecessary or frivolous use of services assumes that people can tell whether that use is necessary or not. Second, it assumes that charges will deter the unnecessary user. Both assumptions are questionable. Many patients are in no position to know whether their symptoms are serious or not. Also, it is often and incorrectly assumed that the only costs of health care are any charges which may be levied by providers. But an important additional cost is time away from other activities which can be very important not only for those who lose cash earnings when away from work but also for subsistence farmers and, not least, for mothers taken away from their household duties. A further cost is that of travel for many patients.

Decisions to seek health care and who to consult depend on many factors – hours of service, travel time, waiting time, perceived seriousness of health problems, the availability of health providers or of drugs and the way patients are treated, but price is also important. Not surprisingly charges will normally reduce the demands on health services and those whose demands are most reduced are likely to be the poorest. If the yield of the charges is successfully used to improve services, the composition of the user population may change. The better-off may switch back to the government health services, disguising a drop in demand by the poorer section of the population. Increasing reliance on direct payments often makes access harder for the poorest and neediest. However, there are also well-documented experiences of where revenue has been governed locally and spent on drugs or salary improvements, this can lead to improved quality of care, leading to increased demand and improved welfare for poor patients.

A fundamental difficulty with any system of charges is how to exempt the poor. The argument that those who can afford it should pay the full cost of the health services they use and that differential fees should be used 'to protect the poor' makes sense, but is often difficult to apply. However, there are examples of non-governmental health provider organizations in particular that are able to do this; they are most successful where their staff has served a community for long periods and the organization has extensive contacts and knowledge about local families. Traditional healers are also able to collect charges, but they also have close links with the community, are often willing to accept payment in kind and wait until resources are available to pay them, for example, in rural communities this may not be until harvest time.

Willingness to pay does not automatically mean ability to pay. People may be able to lay their hands on money rather than face the humiliation of claiming exemption. But this does not mean that they do not go without before the harvest time or before the next pay comes in or later get into a spiral of debt at high rates of interest and even end up by selling some of their land or other essential possessions. In Tanzania it was found that 60 per cent of households had borrowed, pawned or made special sales to pay health care bills. User fees and out-of-pocket payments by consumers of care as the main mechanism for health financing is an inequitable form of financing because it hits the poor hardest and denies people financial protection from catastrophic health expenditure.

Protection against health care costs

A combination of general taxation, social insurance, private health insurance and limited out-of-pocket user charges has become the preferred instrument for health financing in middle- and high-income countries. In these countries, large segments of the population work in urban settings and in formal employment. It is relatively easy to tax such workers at source and to design health systems that are financed by government and/or payroll contributions. Unfortunately, the policy options for financing health care at low-income levels are very restricted. Poor countries often have large populations in the rural and informal sectors, which limits the effective taxation capacity for their governments. In these countries, such populations often have no effective collective arrangements whereby they can pay for health care or obtain protection from the cost of illness.

A related set of problems occurs during the pooling stage of health financing. Pooling requires some transfer of resources from richer to poor, from healthy people to sick people, and from the employed to the economically inactive. Without such pooling, people with little income are exposed to serious financial hardship when they fall ill. Faced with overwhelming demand and very limited resources, governments find it difficult to ration health care so that public expenditure is targeted at the poor. In many poor countries the better-off often benefit more than the poor from public subsidies and public expenditure. Public policies that, in theory, offer health care to the whole population can shunt scarce health care resources away from the poor and towards segments of the population with more political influence over the health care system.

Discouraged by the ability of their governments to reach rural populations and people engaged in the informal sector, communities in poor countries have increasingly been mobilizing themselves to secure financial protection against catastrophic health expenditure. The common feature of community-based health financing schemes is the active involvement of the community in revenue collection, pooling, resource allocation and sometimes, health service provision. Partly guided by the 1994 willingness and ability to pay study in which Helena participated, a community-based health financing scheme was introduced in 1996 in Kwimba district around Sumve hospital in rural North-West Tanzania. It functioned for three years, and appeared to improve financial protection against the cost of illness and allowed better access to essential health care for the participants. However, targets for scaling up beyond around 20,000 participants and achieving financial sustainability were not achieved, and the external donor who had helped to start the scheme stopped the funding. But, was achieving financial sustainability a realistic and even a worthwhile target for which to strive? Helena with her children, and other poorest of the poor could not afford to join the scheme.

Global Health Fund

> *Sustainability is continuously invoked as a key criterion to assess any aid-inducted activity or initiative. Sometimes, the concept is given the weight of a decisive argument. Thus, to declare something 'unsustainable' may sound as equivalent of 'worthless' or even 'harmful', in this way overruling any other consideration.*
>
> Enrico Pavignani and Alessandro Colombo, 2006

Global health defined as a globally shared responsibility for the health of all is not (yet) a broadly accepted concept. There are large differences between the way people living in rich countries practice solidarity for health within their countries, and the way those same people practice solidarity for health beyond the borders of the countries they live in. There remains an enormous gap between rich and poor countries with respect to health spending and health needs. Low- and middle-income countries account for 84 per cent of the global population and 90 per cent of the global disease burden, but only 20 per cent of the global gross domestic product (GDP) and 12 per cent of all health spending. High-income countries spend about a hundred times more on health on a per capita basis than low-income countries: even after adjusting for cost of living differences, rich countries are spending around 30 times more on health. If the inhabitants of rich countries, who spent around 7 per cent of their GDP on public health expenditure, valued their responsibility towards the health of their fellow-countrymen 30 times higher than their responsibility towards the health of people in poor countries, one would expect the equivalent of 0.21 per cent of the GDP of rich countries to be spent on health care for people living in poor countries. Notwithstanding a recent spectacular increase in foreign aid for health – from US$7 billion in 2001 to $21.8 billion in 2007– this is still only 0.05 per cent of the $40,000 billion GDP of rich countries.

It has been estimated that a comprehensive basic package of health care would require a minimum spend of around $50 per capita (at current prices) per year, well above what is being spent now in poor countries on health service delivery. If such an amount is required, then sustainability – in the sense of financial self-sufficiency within the borders of a country– is not realistic in the foreseeable future. It has been estimated that low income countries, whose combined total GDP in 2007 was US$558 billion for 1.0 billion people, or $584 per capita per year, should be able to generate $12–15 per person per year for a basic package of health care, a relatively ambitious – given the current domestic expenditures for health (Tanzania's GDP was $380 and its health expenditure around $9) – but realistic target. This amount would leave a funding gap of $35–38 per person per year or $35–38 billion in total for the one billion people in poor countries.

In conflicts and crisis situations where international medical and humanitarian relief operations are introduced, the issue of financial sustainability is not being considered. This is because medical relief operations are regarded as necessary interventions to help populations get back to where they were before the disaster struck. Peter Piot, the former head of the Joint United Nations Programme on HIV/AIDS, was able to argue successfully that HIV/AIDS should be regarded as a chronic crisis and that countries that are affected by the HIV/AIDS epidemic can be compared with countries emerging from conflict. With this the difference between medical relief and health development became blurred.

Gorik Ooms, the previous director of Médecins Sans Frontières Belgium, argues the case for not aiming for domestic financial sustainability for health care in poor countries. He observes that when the US President's Emergency Plan For AIDS Relief (PEPFAR) was launched by the George W. Bush administration, it contained the word 'relief' in its name. And this was not only because PEPFAR sounds better than PEPFADA – with the last two letters standing for Development Assistance. PEPFAR was conceived as a medical relief programme, not aiming for financial self-reliance within a foreseeable future, but as an emergency response to a crisis. Similarly, the Global Fund to fight AIDS, Tuberculosis and Malaria ('The Global Fund'), does not aim for financial sustainability either anymore: when countries use their Global Fund grants wisely and effectively, they can count on continued support from the Global Fund. The Global Fund has successfully demonstrated the merits of ambitious thinking: the provision of antiretroviral therapy to people living with AIDS, previously dismissed as unsustainable, became widely accepted as soon as the Global Fund provided a long-term funding perspective. In adopting such an approach, the Global Fund is implicitly recognizing access to health and health care as a human right. Foreign assistance, aimed at the human right of health and access to health care as an essential element, is not a matter of charity. Ooms, a lawyer by training, argues that it is a matter of fulfilling international legal obligations.

Recently, articles in the *New York Times*, the *Los Angeles Times*, the *Financial Times* and the *British Medical Journal*, amongst others, have criticized the disease-specific focus of the Global Fund. The Global Fund is under increasing pressure to broaden its mandate and to move away from an approach that does not contribute sufficiently to the achievement of health Millennium Development Goals such as the reduction of maternal and child mortality or beginning to reverse the incidence of diseases other than HIV/AIDS, tuberculosis and malaria, including the chronic non-communicable diseases. Neither does its approach do enough for overall health system strengthening.

So, what about a Global Health Fund that covers a comprehensive basic package of health care? Advantages of such an approach would be that it could provide a means to rationalize the large number of international health aid relationships involving many bilateral agreements as well as single-disease agreements and lead to a harmonization of procedures and increased efficiencies. A single Global Health Fund, to which poor countries would submit their 'package-needs' should then, if adjusted and co-owned by civil society, reflect their real priorities. The pooling could also facilitate civil society taking up responsibility for advocacy and monitoring. Civil society of rich countries could play an important role in mobilizing to push for the generation of the international health aid needed, and civil society in poor countries would have to mobilize to generate increased domestic health financing and to make sure that all health financing is well spent. Civil society in both rich and poor countries should put pressure to end the practice of illegal flight capital – the large sums of money leaving poor countries that escapes the detection of regulatory agencies and ends up on 'safe' bank accounts in rich countries – and advocate that this money is better used for reducing health inequities. Channelling international health aid through a single Global Health Fund could prevent the attachment of political or economic strings. Practices, such as using development assistance to cajole a recipient country into voting a particular way at the United Nations, or providing favourable conditions for the exploitation of their natural resources, would be avoided.

If increased and sustained international aid for health would lead to stagnating or even decreasing domestic health financing, it would limit gains and undermine rich countries' willingness to sustain international health solidarity. The Global Health Fund could demand an agreement with the recipient country and a roadmap towards allocating an increasing amount in-country to the comprehensive basic package of healthcare as a condition for continued international health aid. The Global Health Fund could also help countries to come to an appropriate mix of health financing means that could have country-specific solutions with appropriate combinations of general taxation, social insurance, private health insurance, community health financing schemes including micro-health insurance, and/or limited out-of-pocket user charges for domestic health financing.

Domestic and international pooling, burden sharing and monitoring should also reduce fluctuations in annual health budgets. A single, comprehensive Global Fund would also be in a much stronger position to deal with corruption and misuse of funding than the current system where, with thousands of possible donor funding channels, a new donor often can be found to replace a dissatisfied one. The involvement of civil society can be an important additional 'tool' that can help detect corruption and any misuse of funding.

Another economic crisis

> *I would also like to emphasize the need – the absolute necessity – for us to offer our support to the poorer nations. They are the victims of the crisis. Some now face the real risk of seeing considerable efforts in recent years toward achieving the millennium development goals being completely nullified if we do not show solidarity.*
>
> Nicolas Sarkozy, 2009

In the meantime, the world has become the 'victim' of another economic crisis that is now called the 'economic downturn'. The current financial crisis is affecting people and countries all over the world, rich and poor; and as usual the poor will suffer more than the better-off in the end. Although we are probably not at the end of the crisis, especially for poor countries with a pullback in investment, trade – there has already been another drop in the price of basic commodities – and credit, there seems to be a consensus that the global economic interdependence is a given, and so is the world's increasingly interdependent financial architecture. Even if this financial architecture allowed overconfidence in the market mechanism, and deregulation in some rich countries created the current global crisis, hardly anyone has been seriously considering a return to closed autonomous economies. Government leaders who make statements that reek of protectionism are being criticized immediately by colleagues, economists and the media. That is at least one lesson that seems to have been learned from previous crises. Most governments of rich countries have made statements that they will not reduce international aid. These are hopeful signs. One could argue that a globally shared responsibility to deal with the economic crisis could be expanded to a global responsibility and increased solidarity for global health as one of the adjustments needed to address world poverty and inequity, and a different way of organizing the economy of the planet. Innovative forms of finance include a special airline tax and using this revenue across countries to pool funds and procure through a central mechanism drugs to reduce the market price in poor countries, and the use of tobacco taxes to fund health activities. Swapping existing debt for grants, converting loans to grants with performance targets are other initiatives that could be used and expanded, and can help to fund the strengthening of health systems. Utopian? The ideas put forward here are without any doubt bold, but I would argue that this is the right time to push for the need to strengthen, not weaken, ambitions for alleviating poverty including reducing health inequalities in a global response to the current economic crisis.

Sources and suggestions for further reading

Brian Abel-Smith's *An Introduction to Health Policy, Planning and Financing* (London: Longman, 1994) remains a classic text, and provides an excellent insight into the issues of the 1980s economic crisis, the structural adjustment programmes that followed and its consequences for health financing and health service delivery in poor countries. *Health Financing Revisited: A Practitioner's Guide* by Pablo Gottret and George Schieber (Washington, DC: World Bank, 2006) is a recent comprehensive introduction to health financing that is well-researched, uses a clear and concise writing-style, and provides good information on numerous case studies including from low-income countries. Gorik Ooms' doctoral thesis 'The right to health and the sustainability of health care: Why a new global health aid paradigm is needed' can be found at http:/www.ichr.org/files/academia-doctoraat%20Gorik%20Ooms_0.pdf (accessed 3 March 2009) and is a fascinating and inspiring read on why a comprehensive global health fund makes sense, as well as ideas on how it could be realized. The willingness to pay study in which Helena participated in June 1994 is reported in Gijs Walraven, 'Willingness to pay for district hospital services in rural Tanzania', *Health Policy and Planning* (1996; 11: 428–437), while Alexander Preker et al. report on 'The effectiveness of community health financing in meeting the cost of illness' in the *Bulletin of the World Health Organization* (2002; 80: 143–150). Another review of community health insurance which reveals the major difficulties to be overcome can be found in Manuela De Allegri and others. 'Community health insurance in sub-Saharan Africa: What operational difficulties hamper its successful development? *Tropical Medicine and International Health* (2009; 14: 586–596). The quote by Enrico Pavignani and Alessandro Colombo can be found in module 6 of World Health Organization manual 'Analysing disrupted health sectors: Analysing health sector financing and expenditure', available from http://www.who.int/hac/techguidance/tools/disrupted_sectors/module_6/en/index.html (accessed 24 March 2009), while Nicholas Sarkozy wrote a Global Viewpoint article with the title 'Toward the G-20' that was published in the *International Herald Tribune* of 1 April 2009, and which contained the quote used in this chapter. Reports of the two working groups of a High Level Taskforce, established in

September 2008, on Innovative International Financing for Health Systems, can be accessed at www.internationalhealthpartnership.net/CMS_files/documents/working_group_1_-_report_EN.pdf (this report attempts to address constraints to scaling up and costs) and www.internationalhealthpartnership.net/CMS_files/documents/working_group_2_-_report_EN.pdf (discusses options for raising and channelling funds; both reports accessed 29 January 2010).

12
Cross-border health care

Descending from the 'hidden roof of the World'; its waters tell of forgotten peoples and whisper secrets of unknown lands. They are believed to have rocked the cradle of our race. Long the legendary watermark between Iran and Turan, they have worn a channel deep into the fate of humanity. World-wide conquerors, and Alexander and a Tamerlane, slaked their horses' thirst in the Oxus stream; Eastern poets drank inspiration from its fountains; Arab geographers boasted of it as 'superior in volume, in depth, and in breath to all the rivers of the world'.

George Nathaniel Curzon, 1894

Sanam

I am talking on the phone to Dawlat, whose wife died six months ago. I would have much preferred speaking to him in person, but I have not been allowed to cross the Oxus border river bridge to go to his village, only 3km away from where I am now. I am in Khorog, Tajikistan Badakshan or Gorno-Badakshan, and he is in Bashor, Afghanistan Badakshan. The Tajik–Afghan border has been closed for security reasons in anticipation of a visit by the president of Tajikistan to Gorno-Badakshan. It will remain closed for four days, and during that time no one will be allowed to cross, including any patient needing emergency medical care in Tajikistan that is not available on the other side of the border. And this is the reason why Sanam died in December 2007. She was a healthy 30-year-old woman, mother of two, who died with the history of severe burning abdominal pains, a distended abdomen and not passing stools for three days. Dawlat, who had been looking after Sanam with his mother and father, reported that during these days she could not swallow anything without vomiting it out again. He also felt she had looked pale, and she had complained of chest pain especially during the last day before she died, and the pain had been located over the sternum, and had been continuous. She had been three months pregnant, and had attended antenatal care already once – something that had not been possible with her previous pregnancies as at that time there was no health centre in the area. Dawlat took his wife to the health centre in Bashor on the first day of her illness, where after examination the doctor concluded that she would need to be transferred to a hospital where she might need to have an operation as she was having an 'acute abdomen'. The doctor made enquiries for her transfer to the hospital on the other side of the border – you can see the Khorog hospital from the health centre in Bashor, it really is only separated by the border and the bridge over the Oxus river. In winter especially, in this high mountainous area, Khorog hospital is the only place where patients can be referred to, as the only hospital in Afghanistan Badakshan is then totally inaccessible from the valley where Dawlat lives with his family. The doctor was told by the border guards that the border was closed, and they refused to give permission for crossing. Despite frantic attempts involving authorities on both sides of the border this refusal was upheld until Sanam died on day three of her illness.

The most likely diagnosis, I think, based on the disease history of a woman with classical signs and symptoms of an acute abdomen in early pregnancy (and therefore Sanam's death has to be classified as a maternal death) and severe anaemia, is a ruptured ectopic pregnancy. Intestinal obstruction or perforation are high up in the differential diagnosis. From the history it is also clear to me that Sanam would have had a very good chance to survive and recover fully if she had been able to cross the border and had been stabilized, and had had the abdominal surgery she probably needed.

The lands of the great game

> *Listen to the north, my boys, there's trouble on the wind;*
> *Tramp o' Cossack hooves in front, gray great-coats behind,*
> *Trouble on the Frontier of a most amazin' kind,*
> *Trouble on the waters o' the Oxus!*
>
> Rudyard Kipling, *Soldiers Three*, 1888

> *More people debated the Great Game than ever played it.*
> John Keay, *When Men and Mountains Meet*, 1977

In the high and cold mountainous areas of Central Asia lie the lands that were once contested during the 'Great Game'. This term, 'Great Game', was used to describe the rivalry and strategic conflict between the British and the Russian empire for supremacy in Central Asia. Now, the successor states of the Russian and British empires govern communities in these mountainous areas that are often forgotten and frequently un-served. In some measure, I think that the health status of these communities, and especially of the women and children living in the contiguous border areas of three states (Afghanistan, Pakistan and Tajikistan) reflect the challenges, successes and failures of these states.

Although the communities in these adjacent geographical areas share a common ethnicity, religion and culture, their health indicators vary widely along with the capacities and efforts of governmental and non-governmental actors to reduce the disparities.

In the rural province of Afghan Badakhshan, a remote region with minimal infrastructure and few modern health services, Linda Bartlett and others carried out a reproductive age mortality survey. Reported in 2005, this survey found the highest maternal mortality ratio ever documented (6507 per 100,000 live births) for a three-year time period (April 1999 through to March 2002), and a very high infant mortality rate (217 per 1000 live births). On the other side of the Oxus (Amu Darya, Panji) River sits Gorno-Badakhshan Autonomous Oblast of the newly independent Republic of Tajikistan. Here, the Soviet health system contributed to a relatively low maternal mortality ratio (54 per 100,000 live births) and infant mortality rate (28 per 1000 live births), even as late as 1994. Recent surveys in the Oblast suggest that the new republic's health system has not been able to maintain the indicators achieved during the Soviet period. In the Northern Areas of Pakistan, a disputed territory but contiguous with the other regions, local government institutions have traditionally been very weak. Yet, important improvements in maternal and child health indicators, including a substantial reduction in the maternal mortality ratio (from 550 to 68 per 100,000 live births) and infant mortality rate (from 158 to 31 per 1000 live births) have been observed over the last 20 years. While under-reporting of maternal, infant and especially neonatal deaths is a global problem, and differences in the data collection methods challenge the comparability of the measures across the three regions, the substantial differences strongly suggest true differences that should be examined to determine why women and infants in the Northern Areas and Gorno-Badakshan have a markedly lower risk of death compared to Afghanistan Badakshan.

Maternal and child health in Afghan Badakshan and adjacent cross-border areas

North-Eastern Afghanistan

The challenges facing the Afghanistan health authorities in the province of Badakshan are daunting. The population is extremely poor, largely illiterate and widely dispersed, women's mobility is restricted, and health facilities are few, ill-equipped and staffed by a small number of poorly trained staff (as can be seen in Table 12.1). The Afghan government, with support from international donor agencies, contracted the Aga Khan Development Network (AKDN) to implement a health programme in the province. The programme, which started in 2003, follows the Ministry of Public Health policy that makes a single non-governmental organization responsible for planning, implementing and monitoring the health services in a district or province. This approach attempts to avoid duplication of effort, ensure efficient control of resources and promote effective programme management.

Table 12.1 *Health indicators for Afghanistan and Afghan Badakhshan, Pakistan and Northern Areas, Tajikistan and Gorno-Badakshan*

INDICATOR	Afghanistan		Pakistan			Tajikistan		
	Badakhshan 2004[1]	Afghanistan 2005[2]	Northern Areas 1986[3]	Northern Areas 2004[4]	Pakistan 2005[2]	Gorno Badakshan 1994[3]	Gorno Badakshan 2004[3]	Tajikistan 2005[2]
Population covered by programme	133,000	28.6 m	283,000	312,000	154.8 m	228,000	213,000	6.4 m
Maternal mortality ratio (per 100,000 live births)	6,507	1,900	550	68	500	54	116	59
Infant mortality rate (per 1,000 live births)	217	165	158	31	79	28	38	71
Under-5 mortality rate (per 1,000 live births)	323	257	n.a.	39	99	n.a.	52	100
Life expectancy (yrs)	46	46	53	67	64	n.a.	69	64
Life expectancy: females as a proportion of males	96	101	102	102	101	n.a.	110	109
Contraceptive prevalence (%)	1	10	n.a.	33	28	32	45	34
Skilled attendant at delivery (%)	2	14	13	88	31	70	76	71
1 year old children vaccinated against measles (%)	69	64	11	90	78	40	70	84
Adult literacy rate, female (%)	11	13	9	32	36	n.a.	98	99
Primary school enrolment ratio, female (%)	70	56	13	66	69	n.a.	100	97
% of population using safe water sources	0.3	39	5	58	91	36	36	59
% of population using adequate sanitation facilities	0	34	8	51	59	83	83	51
Number of physicians per 1,000 population	0.1	0.2	n.a.	0.3	0.7	n.a.	2.1	2
Number of nurses per 1,000 population	0.2	n.a.	n.a.	1.6	n.a.	n.a.	8.9	n.a.
Number of hospital beds per 1,000 population	0.2	0.4	n.a.	0.8	0.7	n.a.	9.1	6.1
Annual Gross Average Income per capita (US$)	80	250	132	288	690	n.a.	235	330
Operational costs of the AKDN health programme per capita (in US$)	11.2	n.ap.	n.a.	6.7	n.ap.	1.8	5	n.ap.

n.a. = not available   n.ap. = not applicable
(1) Data on maternal, infant and under five mortality obtained from the Bartlett et al study (2005), other data obtained from specific surveys covering the catchment population using multiple indicator cluster (MICS) and knowledge practice coverage (KPC) modules and methodologies (see www.childinfo.com/mics and www.childsurvival.com/kpc2000)
(2) Data obtained from www.unicef.org/infobycountry (first source) and www.worldbank.org/data/countrydata (second source used for missing data) (both last accessed on 30th November 2007). Note: where 2005 data are not available, table shows nearest available year.
(3) Data obtained from specific surveys covering the catchment population using questionnaires similar to MICS and KPC modules and methodologies (see www.childinfo.org/mics and www.childsurvival.com/kpc2000). For the maternal mortality estimations the reproductive age mortality survey methodology was used.
(4) Demographic data including mortality data obtained from the routine demographic surveillance system in the catchment population, other data obtained from specific surveys.

Health care is provided through a three-tiered system, consisting of:

- community health workers; one woman and one man per community of around 1000 people who are chosen by the community, native to the local area and literate where possible;
- basic health centres with outreach, mainly concentrating on outpatient services and normal deliveries, and covering a population of 5000–10,000; and
- comprehensive referral health centres with inpatient capacity and comprehensive obstetric services that includes the capacity for performing caesarean sections and blood transfusion services, covering a minimum population of 25,000.

At the close of 2009, the system in the Afghanistan Badakshan border districts included 198 community health workers in 99 villages, 17 basic health centres and 3 comprehensive health centres. This network is providing health care to an estimated 157,000 people, and focuses on primary care interventions such as child immunization; micronutrient supplementation and nutrition screening; tuberculosis control; prenatal, delivery and post-partum care; family planning; and basic curative services, including integrated management of childhood illnesses. A community midwifery school, affiliated with the only hospital in the province, has been established. So far 80 graduates, who received 18 months of training including modules on child health care and health promotion and disease prevention, have been posted at health centres closest to their home communities. To bridge the geographical gap in access in this isolated and high mountainous area, the acceptability and feasibility of establishing maternity waiting homes near health facilities have been assessed and based on the positive findings these are being established.

In addition to health services, other interventions are being implemented. Programmes in education (with a major emphasis on female education), natural resource management, agriculture and marketing, water and sanitation infrastructure, road construction, tele-communication, electricity, microfinance, small business development and civil society promotion are combined with economic development and cultural restoration activities to constitute an area development programme. The impact of this approach on reducing maternal and child mortality remains to be determined. Sanam could not yet be helped, but there are promising signs of increases in the availability and utilization of health services between 2004 and 2009.

Northern Pakistan

In the Northern Areas of Pakistan, which is a disputed territory without strong local governmental institutions and currently afflicted with sectarian tensions and only accessible by road and air when the weather is favourable, public sector services have been and remain too limited to reach the great majority of the remote and dispersed rural communities. Over the past 20 years AKDN has developed a three-tiered health system similar to the one introduced in Afghan Badakshan. The community-based model provides outreach through a network of private, not-for-profit health facilities, linked with male and female community health workers who carry out health promotion and disease prevention activities. Communities participate and contribute to the establishment of the health facilities, provide land and labour, and pay (limited) user fees.

Since the 1980s, there have been important improvements in maternal and child health indicators. The community nurse-midwife (called a Lady Health Visitor) plays a key role in the system. These women are the first level health professionals with maternal and child health skills and provide the community health workers with continuing education and supervision, perform maternal and child health care including deliveries both at home and in the health centres, and form the link between village-level primary health care and referral health services. Considerable attention is given to continuing education and supervision, and to ensuring that there is a good enabling environment with correct coordination and organization of services, including supplies, training and communications. The communities, through local health committees, actively support the safety and well-being of the community midwives. To ensure that referrals are timely, the community's capacity to manage complications and to respond to emergencies has been addressed simultaneously with efforts to improve the quality of facility-based health services.

Tajikistan

The Soviet health system contributed successfully to achieving relatively good health status for the communities in Gorno-Badakhshan. At the same time, however, the system in Gorno-Badakshan had an excess number of hospital beds and staff (with an estimated 9 hospital beds, 2 doctors and 16 nurses per 1000 population) (see Table 12.1 and Figure 12.1).

Health facilities and services, once widely available and generously financed by Moscow, became almost non-functional following the break-up of the Soviet Union, the cessation of subsidies and the outbreak of civil war (1992–1997). All public sectors, including health care, were expected to make a transition from a state-run to a more market-oriented system. Over time, the government recognized the need to make structural changes and defined a health reform strategy. To achieve its vision of a sustainable, cost-effective health system accessible to all, the government intends to promote effective public health measures: enhancing primary health care by developing a Family Medicine speciality; reducing duplication and increasing efficiency in the hospital system; building the capacity of health professionals; and involving the community in developing and governing the system.

Maternal and child health interventions in the programme include birth preparedness through the provision of community-level training, and the upgrading and equipping of health facilities; newborn care and treatment

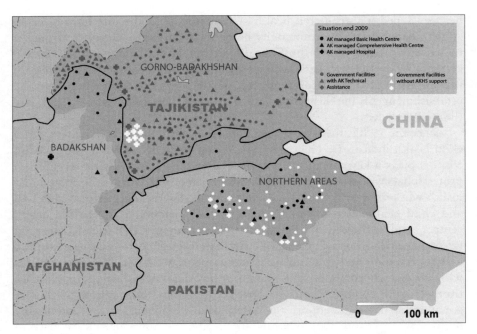

Figure 12.1 *Health facilities in the border districts of Afghan Badakshan, the Northern Areas of Pakistan (now called Gilgit-Baltistan), and Gorno-Badakshan in Tajikistan*

improvement through awareness-raising and training on neonatal care and complications; maternal and young child nutrition through training on breastfeeding, child development and complementary feeding, support for routine growth monitoring and research, testing the feasibility and effectiveness of adopting a home-based food fortification approach that uses 'sprinkles', (sachets containing a combination of vitamins, folic acid, iron and zinc); and household level water supply and sanitation through health and hygiene promotion by community health workers.

Maternal and child health indicators, health systems and difficult environments

The experiences described above are not formal studies, and it is difficult to attribute impact to specific interventions. Moreover, it would be incorrect to attribute the reduction in maternal or infant mortality in the Northern Areas of Pakistan solely to health system interventions. Factors such as a better-educated population, the empowerment of women and improved transportation infrastructure are undoubtedly important. One can argue that a reduction of maternal and infant mortality reflects the combined and complex interplay of factors within health systems, but also in the political, economic, social and cultural spheres. Women's work load, nutritional status, education, access to productive resources and social standing in society are influenced by context-specific gender relations as well as levels and distribution of economic resources. These factors interact with access to care of different quality in the three areas discussed in this chapter and produce very different maternal and infant/child outcomes.

Reducing maternal and child mortality is an immense challenge. This is especially so in 'difficult environments', defined as those where the state is unable to harness domestic and international resources effectively to reduce poverty. Projections indicate that the targets of the global Millennium Development Goals, including the target to reduce by three-quarters the maternal mortality ratio and under-5 mortality rate by two-thirds, cannot be met, regardless of how much progress is made in other poor, but well-governed environments, unless substantial improvement takes place in the many areas of the world that are regarded as 'difficult environments'.

The evidence-base for organizing, delivering and paying for effective and equitable health services in any resource-constrained setting is very weak. To make health service delivery work in difficult environments, such as Afghanistan Badakshan, the Northern Areas in Pakistan and Gorno-Badakshan in Tajikistan, poses substantial challenges because each of these areas have to overcome 'traps', identified by Paul Collier in his engaging and provoking book *The Bottom Billion; Why the Poorest Countries are Failing and What Can Be Done About It*. These traps concern bad governance, emerging from civil war and/or being landlocked. To improve maternal and child health indicators, emphasis must be given to strengthening health systems, increasing access to information and care, and addressing the related community and development issues.

Developing human resources, introducing quality-improvement interventions, and implementing strategies for scaling-up and sustaining interventions have been identified as the top priorities for strengthening health systems in the Northern Areas of Pakistan over the last 20 years, and more recently in Gorno-Badakshan and Afghanistan Badakshan. Going to scale and sustaining maternal and child health programmes in difficult environments is rarely achieved. For example, after 20 years of implementation, the cost-recovery of the Pakistan Northern Areas health programme, with its primary objectives of reducing maternal and child mortality, stands at approximately 50 per cent. Moreover, some success in one part of a programme has increased service expectations, expressed as the demand for health care for non-communicable diseases and accidents, and the provision of services for men and older people. There is, then, a real danger that meeting increased and different demands and needs might undermine the health system and contribute to a levelling off or an increase in maternal and child mortality.

The programme in Afghanistan is implemented within the framework of performance-based partnership agreements, a 'contracting-out model'. The government's Ministry of Public Health has the stewardship role. It contracts non-governmental organizations to provide defined services, and monitors and evaluates the performance of the interventions on the basis of a standard set of indicators. International donors provide funding on a standard per capita basis; this is currently negotiated at US$3–6 per capita (depending on the district and the donor). AKDN's experience indicates that the amount provided only covers approximately 20–50 per cent of real operational costs, calculated as $11.2 per capita. Although a weighting component, which relates to the geographical accessibility of the area to be served, is provided, it is too limited.

In addition to donor funding, modest user fees for services were charged until recently, albeit with many exemptions to protect the poor. Fees and exemption rules were set by the village health committee that also decided on the use of the income. These fees recovered an estimated 4 per cent of total operational costs. In the mid-term, even with an improving local economy, going to scale will depend on securing external funding. At present, Afghanistan does not have enough resources, partly because international donor agencies are not committing financial support beyond the short term. A stronger economic base might be attained by the compound/multiplier effect of the integrated programming and area development approach that is being put in place; still, this will take a long time.

In Tajikistan, and Gorno-Badakshan in particular, the transition from a state- to a more market-oriented system, called for a shift away from centralized public financing, with health care free at the point of delivery, to a more cost-effective system based on a mixed financing model underpinned by social health insurance. In practice, however, the transition has not happened as predicted; the shift was imposed from outside and took place suddenly, leading to a breakdown in the health infrastructure. Financial shortages have triggered a huge increase in out-of-pocket payments, including informal payments to health professionals, who saw their salaries drop to levels below $1 per day, and a concurrent decrease in coverage for the population. A possible way forward could be a carefully planned health insurance schedule that drives the health reform, has systems for monitoring quality of care, and has greater involvement of community and civil society organizations in decision-making. However, this will take time and require all stakeholders to agree on how: (a) contracting relationships will work; (b) to develop regulations that govern these relationships; and (c) to strengthen capacity to implement rules designed to encourage innovation and reduce risk of failure.

The case for 'cross-border health care'

One additional strategy that deserves more attention is an approach based on 'cross-border health care'. Traditionally the borders were porous and people crossed easily and often to visit markets and trade; marriages across the border were common. This changed from the 1930s onwards, when the Tajik border became tightly controlled by Russian border guards and the borders were virtually closed. Following the collapse of the Soviet Union, and with the opening of three bridges over the Oxus River since 2003 at the Afghan–Tajik (Gorno)-Badakshan border, a start has been made to restore some of the former practices that served local community needs. However, to date, maternal and child health programmes in each location have been addressed within the capacities of the states and the civil society institutions. These efforts have produced very different results because the capacities of the key actors vary considerably. Enhancing capacities is a long-term effort but one that must be started immediately, and efforts to promote cross-border collaboration has the potential to lead to quick but sustainable improvements. Our experience shows that recruiting and posting health professionals from Gorno-Badakshan and the Northern Areas of Pakistan, who speak the same language and share a common cultural background, to Afghanistan Badakshan, is possible and acceptable to both health professionals and the local communities. Although it failed with Sanam, it has also been possible to get some critically ill patients from Afghanistan Badakshan treated in Tajik hospitals, and for policy-makers from Gorno-Badakshan and Afghan Badakshan to make study tours to the Northern Areas of Pakistan in order to observe its primary health care system. As confirmed by focus group discussions and in-depth interviews held with health professionals, patients, border authorities and policy-makers, cross-border health care is achievable, but only if it is well-regulated and the regulations are enforced.

A major challenge is to overcome the lack of trust at the level of the central governments, mainly related to cross-border security and narcotics smuggling issues. However, it could be argued that defining an effective cross-border health policy could be a first important step towards building trust. Measures that have not been addressed sufficiently but could greatly increase the chances for success, and recommended by participants in AKDN's qualitative research, include simplification of the border crossing procedures, setting up transparent costing and pricing at a full cost-recovery level of all interventions with agreed financing mechanisms, and adequate communication of the potential benefits for all stakeholders in the different countries.

A 'cross-border health' policy offers the potential to release human and financial resources in all three states, contributing to more rapid progress than can be imagined by the 'conventional routes' because the approach maximizes the use of existing resources. Although not easy to implement, experiences elsewhere – albeit mainly in Europe – have shown that 'regulated' movement of health professionals and patients is possible; moreover, it can improve health care by making use of different capabilities of health care services in different countries.

Poverty has many faces

> *Development requires the removal of major sources of unfreedom: poverty as well as tyranny, poor economic opportunities as well as systematic deprivation, neglect of public facilities as well as overactivity of repressive states. Despite unprecedented increases in overall opulence, the contemporary world denies elementary freedoms to vast numbers of people.*
>
> Amartya Sen, 1999

> *Reducing health inequities is, for the Commission on Social Determinants of Health, an ethical imperative. Social injustice is killing people on a grand scale.*
>
> The World Health Organization Commission on
Social Determinants of Health, 2008

A 'cross-border health policy' can possibly contribute something to the improvements of health indicators across the region, but it is clearly not the panacea for everything. Poverty has many faces; it is being ill and not being able to access health care that should be accessible, and it is losing a child to illness brought about by unclean water, malaria or disease that can be prevented with immunization. Poverty is not having access to school and not knowing how to read. Poverty is not having a job, living with insecurity from day to day. Poverty is being powerless, with a lack of representation and freedom.

Amartya Sen, the 1998 Nobel Prize winner for Economics, defined freedom (which he regards as requisite for development) as an interdependent bundle of political freedom and civil rights, economic freedom, social opportunities, transparency guarantees and protective security. He argued that people's welfare (including arrangements for health care, education and other social services) can be addressed best through a democratic system in which people are able to bring their needs to the fore; and that democratic accountability provides incentives for leaders to deal with issues of broad impact such as health. Large inequities in health within and between countries arise not only from inadequate, and unfair, distribution of health care but are also determined by what are now called the social determinants of health. Marked health inequities between and within countries are caused by the unequal distribution of power, income, goods and services. Gaps in health and health care are not a matter of fate – they are indicators of policy failure. To tackle inequalities in health will need the prioritization and strengthening of primary health care and health systems, as well as a social justice approach to health and greater attention to intersectoral actions – at the global, national and local level.

Sources and suggestions for further reading

Peter Hopkirk's *The Great Game* is a classic work that tells the story of the great imperial struggle for strategic and economic supremacy fought across the region of Central Asia (London: John Murray, 1990), while Paul Garnier's *The Bottom Billion* (Oxford: Oxford University Press, 2007) is a must read for everyone who wants to understand what is happening to the poorest billion in the world, and why it is happening. This book also provides a number of provocative ideas on what can be done to help them. The paper by Linda Bartlett and others referred to in the text, 'Where giving birth is a forecast to death: Maternal mortality in four districts in Afghanistan, 1999–2002', can be found in *The Lancet* (2005; 365: 864–870). For a good account on the issues around scaling up the most important health interventions that can make a difference to poor people see K. Hanson et al., 'Expanding access to priority health interventions: A framework for understanding the constraints to scaling-up', *Journal of International Development* (2003; 15: 1–14). A shorter and earlier version of the case for cross-border health can be found in G. Walraven et al., 'Improving maternal and child health in difficult environments: Experiences in adjacent geographical areas in Afghanistan, Pakistan, and Tajikistan and the case for "cross border" health care', *PLoS Medicine* (2009; 6: e5). In *Development as Freedom* (New York: Knopf, 1999), Amartya Sen defines and elaborates on development as 'the enhancement of freedoms that allow people to lead lives that they have reason to value'. The final report of the Commission on Social Determinants of Health, 'Closing the gap in a generation: Health equity through action on the social determinants of health', can be downloaded for free from the World Health Organization's website: www.who.int/social_determinants/final_report (last accessed 10 October 2009).

13

Revisiting Alma Ata

I am now convinced that we will not be able to reach the health-related Millennium Development Goals unless we return to the values, principles, and approaches of primary health care.

Margaret Chan, 2007

More than 30 years ago, in the midst of the Cold War, health experts and policy makers from 134 countries convened in a city in what is now Kazakhstan, to attend a conference on international primary health care. On 12 September 1978, the Alma Ata Declaration was signed, with the ambitious goal of achieving 'health for all' by the year 2000. Alma Ata's target of 'health for all' was based on the World Health Organization's constitutional definition, where health is 'a state of physical, mental and spiritual well-being, not merely an absence of disease or infirmity' – a highly aspirational rather than measurable objective. According to Hafdan Mahler, the inspirational director-general of the World Health Organization at the time, Alma Ata was 'one of the rare occasions where a sublime consensus between the haves and the have-nots in local and global health emerged'. Its Declaration revolutionized the world's interpretation of health with the core principles of universal access to care, equity, community participation, intersectoral collaboration, and appropriate use of resources, as well as by stating that inadequate and unequal health care was unacceptable: economically, socially and politically. Box 13.1 shows the description of primary health care in the declaration. With an emphasis on local ownership, primary health care honoured the resilience and ingenuity of the human spirit and made space for solutions created, owned and sustained by communities. Primary health care also offered a way to organize the full spectrum of health care, from households to hospitals, with prevention as important as cure, and with resources invested rationally in the different levels of care.

Unfortunately, the goal of 'health for all' by the year 2000 was not met. When asked about the meaning of the 'health for all' goal, Hafdan Mahler said 'the goal was not to eradicate all diseases and illnesses by 2000; we knew that would have been impossible. Our goal was to focus world attention on health inequalities and on trying to attain an acceptable level of health, equitably distributed throughout the world.'

Box 13.1 *Description of Primary Health Care from the Alma Ata Declaration*

1 Reflects and evolves from economic conditions and sociocultural and political characteristics of the country and its communities, and is based on application of relevant results of social, biomedical and health-services research and public-health experience.
2 Addresses main health problems in the community, providing promotive, preventative, curative and rehabilitative services accordingly.
3 Includes at least: education about prevailing health problems and methods of preventing and controlling them; promotion of food supply and proper nutrition; adequate supply of safe water and basic sanitation; maternal and child health care, including family planning; immunization against major infectious diseases; prevention and control of locally endemic diseases; appropriate treatment of common diseases and injuries; and provision of essential drugs.
4 Involves, in addition to the health sector, all related sectors and aspects of national and community development, in particular, agriculture, animal husbandry, food, industry, education, housing, public works, communications, and other sectors; and demands coordinated efforts of all those sectors.
5 Requires and promotes maximum community and individual self-reliance and participation in planning, organization, operation, and control of primary health care, making fullest use of local, national, and other available resources; and to do this develops, through appropriate education, ability of communities to participate.
6 Should be sustained by integrated, functional and mutually supportive referral systems, leading to progressive improvement of comprehensive health for all, and giving priority to those most in need.
7 Relies, at local and referral levels, on health workers, including physicians, nurses, midwives, auxiliaries, and community health workers as applicable, as well as traditional practitioners as needed, suitably trained socially and technically to work as a health team and to respond to expressed health needs of the community.

In addition, the comprehensive approach of Alma Ata was almost immediately misunderstood; it was regarded by some as an attack on the medical establishment, and it was confused with an exclusive focus on first-level health care. For some it was regarded as cheap: poor care for poor people, a second rate solution for poor countries. And within a year of the Declaration, a simpler approach was proposed involving a more top-down approach and focusing on a few interventions most justified by epidemiological importance and technical affordability. This more selective approach was considered to be more feasible, measurable, rapid, and less risky than really empowering communities to make choices. These interventions, such as immunization, family planning and micronutrients were delivered through 'vertical' programmes, which took the decisions out of the hands of communities, but rapidly reached high coverage for the selected priorities. The emergence of HIV, the associated resurgence of tuberculosis and an increase in malaria strengthened the move towards the selective management of priority diseases and high-mortality emergencies. The health-related Millennium Development Goals were developed in line with this selective approach. And while the Millennium Development Goals set ambitious targets, including in the health sector, they said little or nothing about the delivery. Primary health care was hardly mentioned in the Millennium Declaration.

As argued in this book, progress towards the Millennium Development Goals so far has been insufficient. Weak health care systems have restricted the success of efforts to improve maternal, newborn and child health, and to reduce the disease burden from AIDS, tuberculosis and malaria. New epidemics of chronic diseases, both of infectious (including AIDS, although it is still largely managed as an acute illness) and non-communicable origin such as cardiovascular diseases, diabetes, mental diseases and cancer (although especially in poor countries often with an infectious cause), threaten to reverse what small gains have been achieved. In addition, there are other emerging challenges of increasing numbers of injuries and other health risks associated with urbanization and globalization, including the threat of pandemics, the trade in harmful products such as tobacco, alcohol and other drugs, the health consequences of climate change, and the dissemination of harmful lifestyle practices.

The 2008 World Health Report, entitled *Primary Health Care: Now More than Ever*, states that international and national policy formulation processes continue to focus on single issues, with many constituencies competing for increasing but still scarce resources, while little attention is given to addressing constraints to health systems development. Rather than improving their response capacity and anticipating new challenges, health systems seem to be drifting from one short-term priority to another, increasingly fragmented and without a clear sense of direction. To accelerate progress to be able to meet the Millennium Development Goals by 2015, countries need to strengthen their health systems through the implementation of effective primary health care.

What can be learned from the Alma Ata primary health care movement?

> *Health for all need not be a dream buried in the past.*
> Lancet Editorial, 2008

Today, primary health care is no longer so poorly understood. The evidence that countries with a strong emphasis on primary health care have better outcomes at low cost is strong. Countries that have achieved meaningful progress in health indicators include Thailand, Vietnam, Peru, Nepal, Bangladesh and Kazakhstan. Common features of these countries include accountable leadership, the training of a skilled workforce including community health workers, community and family participation and ownership, a district level focus and a priority given to equity by removing financial barriers to the poorest families. Essential characteristics of a strong health system led by primary health care include good accessibility and no financial barriers, a person (not disease) focus over time, a broad range of services in primary care, and coordination when people need to be referred for higher level care. The key to 'success' countries often was: national essential health packages with defined priorities and links to the not-for-profit sector, non-governmental organizations, and other service providers in the system.

The Millennium Development Goals have re-emphasized the values of equity and social justice, important in 'Alma-Ata'. The chronic diseases epidemics bring new challenges with the burden of long-term care on already stretched health systems and budgets, and costs that can drive households deeper into poverty. This comes with a need for fairness and efficiencies. There is a clear need for increased efforts towards prevention, but most risk factors are outside the direct control of the health sector. This asks for multisectoral action and community participation.

There is good evidence to support task shifting or task sharing, by which tasks in the health system delivery are allocated to the least costly health worker capable of doing that task reliably. Community health workers can very well assess, classify and manage episodes of routine childhood illnesses, and counsel children's carers. Midwives can be trained in manual vacuum aspiration to control uterine bleeding, trained nurses and medical assistants can do minor surgery, and assistant medical officers can perform caesarean sections safely. Often these initiatives are resisted by professional bodies. If this blocks the delivery of effective essential care to remote populations, they may be seen to promote the narrow economic interests of specific professional groups and lose the trust of the public.

New and emerging technologies can make great contributions to reduce the burden of disease, although it must be emphasized that primary health care is more than a simple summation of individual technological solutions. Insecticide-treated bed nets and artemisinin combination treatments for malaria; oral misoprostol or 'uniject' oxytocin for the prevention of post-partum haemorrhage in home births; pneumococcal, hepatitis B, *Haemophilus influenza* type b and HPV vaccines; vitamin A and zinc supplementation in early childhood; DOTS for tuberculosis; neglected tropical diseases drugs, and a simple multi-drug regimen of aspirin, blood pressure-lowering drugs, cholesterol-lowering drugs and health promotion advice for individuals at high risk of cardiovascular disease are some examples. Also of great importance are recent developments in telecommunications such as mobile phones, which allow patients to be diagnosed and treated in a rural primary health care centre by a provider working in a high-specialty urban hospital. Appropriate technologies should no longer be identified with primitive methods. A related transformation means moving beyond health facilities, which by definition concentrate human and technological resources into health spaces, to promote the reach of comprehensive primary health care into schools, workplaces, recreational areas and the homes of those who live with a chronic condition.

Primary health care: now more than ever

We have invested disproportionally in a form of medicine ('Band Aid' salvage) whose benefits often come late, which buy a little time, and which are easily nullified by external, countervailing factors. Curative, interventionist medicine has played a modest part in shaping wider morbidity and mortality patterns within the community, but in terms of its professed aims – the greatest health of the greatest number – the Olympian verdict must be that much medicine has been off target.

Roy Porter, *The Greatest Benefit to Mankind*, 1997

In a well-functioning health system there are health promotion and prevention activities at the community level, and a patient will go in the first instance to a primary health care centre. Only if that clinic lacks the skills and equipment to treat the patient will they go to a next level of health service delivery, and the same applies for further levels. The system is advantageous for the patient and relatives, as primary health care facilities can be small and therefore within reasonable travel distance. This system is also economical because it should lead to expensive skills and equipment being used only on patients who need it. If a patient who should have been treated at a first level referral community or district hospital is admitted to a next level referral care hospital, more expensive diagnostic tests are likely to be used to confirm the diagnosis of a common condition, simply because the facilities are available.

In practice, and particularly in poor countries this system often does not work as intended. A high proportion of patients treated in hospital could have been treated in a primary health care centre. This is partly because the patient knows that the hospital has better facilities and has doctors with specialized skills. The patient thus goes direct to its outpatient department in the hope of the 'best' treatment, bypassing primary care. It may also happen because it is known that the hospital hardly ever runs out of supplies, particularly of drugs, while this is often the case at lower levels of the health care system. Thus hospitals become used by local, often more affluent urban patients with common conditions. And the costs of treating these common conditions are much higher at the hospital than they would have been at a primary health care clinic.

High tech medicine reflects a period of steady progress since the beginning of the 20th century. For almost all diseases something can now be done, and many diseases can be cured. However, although we have learned more and more about the minutiae of how these diseases make patients sick, we have not made enough headway in determining why they arise in the first place. And much of the progress in their symptomatic management has been achieved by the development of increasingly expensive 'patch-up' procedures. Given the ingenuity of the medical sciences and the pharmaceutical industry, there is no reason why we should not go on improving our ability to repair our patients and extend their lives. But should this be the only goal, and also, can we afford to go on this way? In recent years some serious international rethinking of these questions has taken place. Much of this has been generated by the simple reality that not even the richest countries can find a way of coping with the spiralling costs of health care. Furthermore, there is increasing evidence that many common diseases are related to behaviour, lifestyle and environments.

Many of the ills of health care systems reflect an overreliance on advanced medical technology and an overestimation of the benefits of cure, rather than prevention of disease or the promotion of health. Worrisome trends include health systems that focus disproportionally on a narrow band of specialized curative care, and where a hands-off approach to governance has allowed unregulated commercialization of health care to flourish. There is increasing support for a renewal of efforts to put primary health care at the centre of the overall health system; this springs from the realization among health policy-makers that primary health care can provide a stronger direction and unity in the current context of fragmentation.

The challenge: primary health care and health systems

> *In our age, the greatest challenge before world medicine is to see that the most useful parts of the knowledge we already have are brought to all those who need it.*
>
> Maurice King, 1975

Funding for development assistance for health has quadrupled from US$5.6 billion in 1990 to $21.8 billion in 2007. A worldwide outcry around the turn of the millennium over the plight of people in poor countries especially those in Africa dying of AIDS, a disease kept in check in affected people in rich countries with drugs, triggered a rush to fund big global disease-fighting programmes. On the plus side, millions of people are alive because of the roll-out of HIV drugs to more than 4 million people in poor countries. Coverage of antiretroviral drugs for the prevention of mother-to-child transmission in HIV-positive pregnant women in poor countries increased from 9 per cent in 2004 to 33 per cent in 2007. The number of children protected against malaria by insecticide impregnated bed nets rose almost eightfold from 3 per cent in 2001 to 23 per cent in 2006. The rate of detection of new cases of tuberculosis rose to 56 per cent in 2006, continuing an upward trend that began in 2002 after several years hovering at 40–50 per cent. Disease elimination programmes, such as for polio, are making reasonably good progress. Global immunization has also made important strides. Some of these programmes have had a wider impact than their immediate focus. For example, following a large injection of funds for HIV/AIDS to Botswana, infant mortality dropped and life expectancy increased for the first time in decades. Data from Rwanda show a significant correlation between HIV interventions and improved antenatal care services and family planning. In Kenya, the distribution of free insecticide-treated bed nets to pregnant women through antenatal care clinics was shown to increase the use of regular services at antenatal care services.

Health care in poor countries was in a bad state before the big influx of money to fight diseases began. Decades of neglect and insufficient investment had weakened health systems in most poor countries. In the 1980s and 1990s economic crises, debt repayment, civil and political unrest, poor governance and environmental pressures exacerbated poverty and inequality in many poor countries, especially in sub-Saharan Africa. Structural adjustment policies that were designed to improve the stability of fragile economies led, in many cases, to cuts in public health spending. Moreover, the globalization of labour markets, gathering pace during the 1990s, increased the emigration of health workers from poor countries that had invested in their training. The worldwide HIV epidemic further damaged health systems that were already overstretched.

The influx of money, programmes and partners to fight diseases was a help but also a burden on health systems, whose weakness at the time hampered the progress of the disease-combating initiatives. To strengthen health systems we need integration between interventions, especially where a collection of distinct vertical programmes exists, and the integration of primary health care with the rest of the system. What is also needed is setting explicit priorities and entitlements through the introduction of a set of guaranteed benefits for all, which are translated into packages of essential health services. These packages can combine the vertical focus on explicit disease priorities with a horizontal strengthening of the health system. Afghanistan is a good example of a country that has seen substantial improvements in its coverage of basic health services in the more secure areas of the country by doing exactly this.

Health systems should be seen not only in terms of their component elements (e.g. human resources, financing, primary care centres, hospitals and technologies), but also in terms of their interrelations. Health systems constitute a set of structured relations between institutions and populations. Often, only the institutional or supply side of health systems is analysed. However, the population is more than a possible beneficiary of the system; it needs to be an essential part of it. Individuals, families and communities have crucial roles to play as patients requiring care, and as consumers with expectations about the way in which they are treated. There needs to be mutual trust, respect and value between the community and health services workers. The earlier mentioned explicit entitlements through the introduction of a set of guaranteed benefits for all, can contribute through empowering people to exercise their right to health care. They are also participating as payers of user fees, taxes, premiums, and therefore as an important source of health financing. As citizens they should have the right to demand access to care, information about health-related issues and accountability from public officials. But they also bear responsibility in their role of, what Julio Frenk, the former Minister of Health of Mexico, calls 'co-producers' of health through therapeutic compliance and health-promoting behaviours. Community participation has now been assessed with rigorous designs and has been shown to improve neonatal mortality in Nepal and India. This reflects one of the core principles of the Alma Ata definition of primary health care emphasizing community participation. Civil society organizations can play an important role in monitoring for good governance and increasing responsiveness to community health priorities.

'New' primary health care should promote major shifts in the relationship between providers and populations. Rather than being reactive to demand, providers should be proactive to health needs by anticipating risks in 'their' populations. This is a major difference between a narrow view of first-level 'contact' health services and the broader perspective of primary health care. Unfortunately, since Alma Ata, the balance has tilted towards personal health care at the expense of population health. Health care of the person should take into account the influences and context of the community. An orientation to the population requires the facility-based primary health care worker to understand the local health problems and their social determinants, plan the most effective preventative and therapeutic interventions for the community, and advocate for improved living conditions, while still providing individual health care. Community health workers can help, and play a vital role in such a primary health care system, especially if they work in tandem with facility-based health staff. And, in contrast to the past, there is now robust evidence, including from Uganda and Pakistan, which shows that community health workers can (a) serve as a bridge between the community and the facility-based primary health care worker and the formal health system; and (b) deliver several interventions, especially for conditions such as acute respiratory infections, malaria, perinatal care and neonatal sepsis. In most settings, these interventions are cost-effective. Some programmes, especially in Asia, have been scaled up to reach large populations.

The institutional side of the health care system also requires new thinking. Much emphasis is being put on decentralizing authority in the health care system to the district level. The idea behind this was that the district level can be more sensitive than central government administration to the needs of local people, and can encourage community participation. Decentralization should be able to provide national policy-makers with information on the progress and problems encountered in the implementation of policies and could encourage intersectoral cooperation for the promotion of health where motivation can be greatest. As stated in a 1988 World Health Organization document, it is the district where 'top down and bottom up meet, if they meet at all'. To be able to 'meet', the district should have a large enough unit of capable supporting technical and managerial staff. Policies can then be adapted, thus making them more responsive and relevant to the local needs and circumstances, flexibility can be fostered, community participation can be enhanced, innovation and creativity can be initiated and tried out without having to be enacted for a whole country. This, however, is textbook language and the reality is still different.

One of the main reasons for the failure of decentralization in many poor countries has been a weakening of the role of the Ministry of Health in its capacity to effectively coordinate the health units, services and resources. There has often been a lack of clear organizational structures and lines of authority, with insufficient analysis to understand the complexity of decentralization. Districts can set out their health care needs, but decisions will be influenced by the availability of funds, by national and provincial priorities, by the skills of those at the central level, and by considerations of equity and other issues. An essential element of health systems strengthening is to better enable Ministries of Health in their stewardship role. This stewardship role at the central level is also of great importance in intersectoral interventions. Strong Ministries of Health are needed to promote health policies. Examples of policies that need agreement from other ministries include road safety measures to prevent traffic accidents, combat tobacco and alcohol consumption, norms to promote occupational health and prevent work-related injuries and education policies to promote gender equity.

The World Health Organization estimates the global deficit of trained health workers to be more than 4 million, and Africa, that has 25 per cent of the world's disease burden, has only 1.3 per cent of the health care providers. Overall, a strong positive correlation exists between health workforce density and health outcomes, indicating the importance of the health workforce for the health of populations. The greatest challenge for new primary health care is the workforce. Requirements include training at all levels with strong managerial components alongside technical proficiency, appropriate supervision, development of teamwork and implementation of incentives to good performance. A major challenge that was not as prevalent 30 years ago as it is today, is the drain of health professionals from poor countries. The consequences of this process are considerable. The international debate around the responsibilities of all participants has produced various proposals, which include the improvement of employment conditions and the development of enabling environments for professional growth in poor countries, the increase in educational investments in both poor and rich countries, and the design of ethical recruitment guidelines.

Although funding for global health has expanded over the last two decades, it remains insufficient, largely short-term, poorly coordinated and unpredictable. The failure of rich countries to fulfil their pledges, and the failure of poor countries to invest sufficiently in health are important barriers to health systems development. Using coverage targets in some global health initiatives to assess activities and distribute funds might encourage a concentration of resources in urban health activities and easily accessible populations, and so contribute to inequity. At the same time, current funding for health does address issues of global importance, but whether they serve the specific health needs of poor countries in the best way possible is not known. Some disbursements in countries with a low disease burden indicate a tendency towards supply-induced demand. For example, in Burkino Faso, where the national HIV prevalence rate in adults aged 15–49 is at a relatively low 1.6 per cent, diagnostic tests for HIV were found to be more frequently available in rural clinics than a basic test for anaemia (haemoglobin). In addition, vertically oriented and externally funded services interfere with the responsibility of the state in its ability to improve its own health services.

The increase in funding for development assistance for health, with increases in domestic spending on health in most poor countries is encouraging. However, the achievement of comprehensive primary health care will require continued growth in international and national sources of funding for many years. At a national level, in addition to defined targets for health, such as those agreed in 2001 in Abuja, Nigeria, where African Heads of State committed themselves to devoting a minimum of 15 per cent of government funds to the health sector, long-term financing strategies for health are needed. These strategies should emphasize methods for pre-payment and be responsive to the comprehensive needs and expectations of populations. Guaranteed protection against the financial consequences of disease is needed. Therefore, risks must be aggregated to protect families from poverty shocks caused by health events. Although community-health insurance is a step in the right direction, we cannot merely promote solidarity among poor people. Rather, we should strive for universal schemes, perhaps the Global Health Fund as discussed in Chapter 11, which promotes fair financing across all groups in society. In addition, incentives for both providers and users need to change. 'New' primary health care should introduce innovations in payment schemes that reward high quality care and responsiveness to the legitimate expectations of individuals, families and communities. Families themselves can benefit from incentives towards health-promoting behaviours, as exemplified by the successful conditional cash transfer programmes implemented in many countries, which have reduced poverty while improving educational, nutritional and health outcomes. National health financing strategies should be developed in a way in which there is no risk of external investment preventing or being substituted for domestic investment. With the extent of the shortfalls in essential investments in health in many poor countries, the global public health community needs to recognize that the contribution of more resources is imperative, despite the current economic situation.

The present interest by major global health actors in strengthening health systems offers a unique opportunity. We have to take advantage of this opportunity to revitalize primary health care for the 21st century. We should leave behind the ideological debates of the past and focus instead on developing primary health care networks that are seamlessly integrated into the overall health system. The vision is thus to assure that high-quality services are provided on the basis of a defined population, through proactive strategies, favouring continuity of care and focused attention for disease prevention and health promotion, guaranteeing an explicit and affordable set of entitlements, and assuring universal protection in health. Therein may lie the key to finally unlocking the full potential of Alma Ata, and reach 'health for all', including, and especially, the poor.

Sources and suggestions for further reading

The original declaration of the International Conference on Primary Health Care held in Alma Ata, USSR from 6 until 12 September 1978 can be found on the webpage http://www.who.int/hpr/NPH/docs/declaration_almata.pdf (accessed 18 July 2009). For the writing of this chapter I made extensive use of the 13 September 2008 special issue on primary health care in The *Lancet*, the World Health Organization's *2008* World Health Report, *Primary Health Care: Now More Than Ever*, and Julio Frenk's paper on 'Reinventing primary health care: The need for health systems integration' in *The Lancet* (2009; 374: 170–173), as well as the article by the World Health Organization collaborative group maximizing positive synergies with the title 'An assessment of interactions between global health initiatives and country health systems', also published in *The Lancet* (2009; 373: 2137–2169). The interview with Hafdan Mahler, the director-general of the World Health Organization from 1973 until 1988 on primary health care and Alma Ata can be found in the *Bulletin of the World Health Organization* (2008; 86: 747–748). Thailand, which had a very high reduction in child mortality of 8.5 per cent per year for the period 1990–2006, committed itself early on to comprehensive primary health care, while also making progress in addressing inequity. Viroj Tangcharoensathien and others have written a very good case study with lessons learned from the Thai experience, commissioned by the health systems knowledge network of the WHO commission on social determinants of health (Geneva: World Health Organization, 2007). Cuba has, with 78 years, the second highest average life expectancy at birth in the Americas, and it has achieved these results despite significant economic difficulties. Under the provoking title 'Thomas McKeown, meet Fidel Castro: Physicians, population health and the Cuban paradox' (*Healthcare Policy* 2008; 3: 21–32), Robert Evans describes how some of the major principles of comprehensive primary health care – integration of personal and community health care, development of human resources for health, and intersectoral cooperation – have had a major role in achieving this success.

Glossary

The glossary provides brief reminders about the meanings of the more technical terms used more than once in the course of the book. Words used only once and explained in their context are not always included here.

Acid-fast bacilli (AFB) – bacteria that retain certain dyes after being washed in an acid solution. Most acid-fast organisms are mycobacteria. When AFB are seen on a stained smear of sputum or other clinical specimen, a diagnosis of tuberculosis should be suspected. If possible, the diagnosis should be confirmed by growing a culture that identifies it as *M. tuberculosis*.

Acute abdomen – a serious abdominal condition characterized by sudden onset, pain, tenderness and muscular rigidity, and often requiring emergency surgery.

African trypanosomiasis – also called African sleeping sickness, is a systemic (bodywide) disease caused by a parasite of the *Trypanosoma brucei* family and transmitted by the bite of the tsetse fly.

AIDS (Acquired Immune Deficiency Syndrome) – a disease caused by a retrovirus, Human Immunodeficiency Virus (HIV), and characterized by failure of the immune system to protect against infections and certain cancers.

Anaemia – a shortage in the number of circulating red blood cells and/or quantity of haemoglobin, leading to an inability to carry oxygen around the body. Symptoms include weakness, lethargy, paleness and breathlessness. Malaria mainly causes anaemia through rupture of red blood cells during merozoite release.

Anopheles – a genus of mosquito, some species of which can transmit human malaria.

Appendicitis – inflammation of the appendix, the small worm-like projection from the first part of the colon.

Artemisinin – a drug used against malaria, derived from the Qinghao plant, *Artemisia annua*.

Arteriosclerosis – a chronic disease characterized by abnormal thickening and hardening of the arterial walls with resulting loss of elasticity.

Ascaris (lumbricoides) – common roundworm infecting human intestines.

Infestation can cause morbidity, and sometimes death, by compromising nutritional status, affecting cognitive processes, inducing tissue reactions and provoking intestinal obstruction or rectal prolapse.

Atherosclerosis – a form of arteriosclerosis in which the inner layers of the artery walls become thick and irregular due to deposits of cholesterol and other fats. This build-up is called 'plaque'.

Autopsy – post-mortem examination of the body to determine the cause of death.

Bacillus Calmette-Guérin (BCG) – a vaccine against tuberculosis that is prepared from a strain of the attenuated (weakened) live bovine tuberculosis bacillus, *Mycobacterium bovis*, which has lost its virulence in humans by being specially cultured in an artificial medium for years.

Beriberi – disease caused by deficiency of thiamine (vitamin B1) and characterized by impairment of the nerves and heart. Symptoms include a feeling of numbness and weakness in the limbs and extremities, loss of appetite and general lassitude, and digestive irregularities.

Birth rate (or crude birth rate) – the number of live births per 1000 population in a given year.

Body mass index – a measure of body fat that is the ratio of the weight of the body in kilograms to the square of its height in meters.

Buruli ulcer – a disfiguring skin disease caused by infection with *Mycobacterium ulcerans*. It is believed that the *M. ulcerans* bacteria cause Buruli ulcers by producing a unique chemical toxin that is destructive to the skin and the underlying tissue.

Carrying capacity – the maximum sustainable size of a resident population in a given ecosystem.

Case-control study – a study that compares two groups of people: those with the disease or condition under study (cases) and a very similar group of people who do not have the disease or condition (controls). Researchers study the medical and lifestyle histories of the people in each group to learn what factors may be associated with the disease or condition.

CD4 cell count – a measurement of the number of CD4 cells in a sample of blood. The CD4 count is an important indicator of the health of the immune system and the progression of HIV infection. A CD4 cell count is used by health care providers to determine when to begin anti-HIV treatment, and to measure response to treatment. Although very variable, a healthy adult has 600–1200 CD4 cells per mm^3 compared with < 200 cells per mm^3 in AIDS patients who require treatment.

Cephalo-pelvic disproportion – the term given when the size, presentation and position of the baby's head in relation to the mother's pelvis prevents dilation of the cervix and/or descent of the baby's head.

Cerebral malaria – this grave complication of malaria happens when infected red blood cells obstruct blood circulation in the small blood vessels of the brain. The complication has a fatality rate of 15 per cent or more, even when treated.

Cervical dysplasia – abnormal cell growth in the cervix that is considered precancerous.

Chagas disease – a type of trypanosomiasis, common in Central and South America, caused by a parasite (*Trypanosoma cruzi*) that is carried by insects known as reduviid bugs, and characterized by the eventual invasion and deterioration of cardiac, gastrointestinal and nervous tissue.

Chloroquine – a drug used for many years against malaria. A very safe and inexpensive drug, but its value has been greatly compromised by the emergence of chloroquine-resistant malaria parasites, in particular, *P. falciparum.*

Cholera – a devastating disease caused by the bacterium *Vibrio cholera.* The symptoms are intense vomiting and extreme watery diarrhoea leading to dehydration, which, unless immediately treated, may be fatal. The key to treating cholera is prompt and complete replacement of the fluid and salt lost through the profuse diarrhoea.

Cholesterol – a waxy, fat-like substance used by the body to build cell walls. It is either produced by the liver or absorbed from the animal fats we eat. Cholesterol is carried in the blood stream by particles called lipoproteins.

Chronic bronchitis – inflammation and swelling of the lining of the airways that lead to narrowing and obstruction of the airways. The inflammation stimulates the production of mucus (sputum), which can cause further obstruction of the airways. Obstruction of the airways, especially with mucus, increases the likelihood of bacterial lung infections.

Civil society – individuals and groups, organized or unorganized, who interact in the social, political and economic domains. Civil society offers a dynamic, multilayered wealth of perspectives and values, seeking expression in the public sphere. Civil society organizations are the multitude of associations around which society organizes itself and which represent a wide range of interests and ties. These can include community-based organizations, indigenous people's organizations and non-governmental organizations.

Cohort study – a prospective study that compares a particular outcome (such as lung cancer) in groups of individuals who are alike in many ways but differ in a certain characteristic (for example, doctors in Britain who smoke compared with those who do not smoke).

Coitus interruptus – sexual intercourse deliberately interrupted by withdrawal of the penis from the vagina prior to ejaculation.

Colposcopy – an examination of the cervix, vagina and surrounding tissues with a special microscope called the colposcope. The purpose of the colposcopy is to detect abnormal cell changes.

Computerized axial tomography (CAT) scan – pictures of structures within the body created by a computer that takes the data from multiple X-ray images that turns them into pictures on a screen. The CAT scan can reveal some soft tissue and other structures that cannot be seen in conventional X-rays.

Conjunctivitis – inflammation of the conjunctiva – the membrane that lines the inner surface of the eyelid. It may be caused by a virus, bacteria, irritating substances or allergens. Symptoms include redness of the eye, increased tears, discharge, itching eyes, burning eyes, blurred vision and sensitivity to light.

Cryotherapy – treatment for cervical dysplasia where the abnormal tissue is frozen to destroy it, using compressed carbon dioxide (CO_2) or nitrous oxide (N_2O) as the coolant. Cryotherapy is regarded as the most practical treatment approach for most low-resource settings given its simplicity and low cost.

Cytology – the study of the microscopic appearance of cells, especially for the diagnosis of abnormalities and cancer.

Death rate (or crude death rate) – the number of deaths per 1000 population in a given year.

Demographic transition – the historical shift from high fertility and mortality to low levels in a population. The decline in mortality usually precedes the decline in fertility, thus resulting in rapid population growth during the transition.

Dengue – infectious disease caused by a virus (genus *Flavivirus*). It is transmitted by mosquitoes in tropical and subtropical climates. It is characterized by high fever, severe headaches and pain in muscles and joints. Dengue haemorrhagic fever (fever, abdominal pain, vomiting, bleeding) is a potentially lethal complication of dengue, affecting mainly children.

Diabetes mellitus – a chronic disease associated with abnormally high levels of sugar (glucose) in the blood. Diabetes is due to two mechanisms: (1) inadequate production of insulin (see below) or (2) inadequate sensitivity of cells to the action of insulin. The two main types of diabetes correspond to these two mechanisms and are called insulin-dependent (type 1) and non-insulin dependent (type 2).

Diarrhoea – loose, watery and frequent bowel movements (three or more stools over a 24-hour period is often used as a definition), often associated with an infection.

Direct causes of maternal mortality – those deaths resulting from obstetric complications of the pregnant state (pregnancy, labour and post-partum), from interventions, omissions, incorrect treatment or from a chain of events resulting from any of the above.

Directly Observed Therapy, Short course (DOTS) – is watching the patient take his/her medication to ensure that the medication is taken in the right combination and for the correct duration. It is used for diseases such as tuberculosis and HIV to assure compliance and avoid drug resistance.

Diverticulitis – inflammation of the diverticula (small outpouches) from the large intestine, the colon.

DNA – Deoxyribonucleic acid. The molecules inside cells that carry genetic information and pass it on from one generation to the next.

Drug resistance – the result of microbes changing in ways that reduce or eliminate the effectiveness of drugs, chemicals or other agents to cure or prevent infections.

Dysentery – a severe intestinal infection, causing abdominal pain and diarrhoea with blood or mucus.

Ectopic pregnancy – a pregnancy that develops outside the uterus, most frequently in one of the fallopian tubes. An ectopic pregnancy can rupture through the tissue in which it has implanted, producing haemorrhage (bleeding) from exposed vessels.

Elimination – reduction to zero of the incidence of locally transmitted infection in a defined geographical area as a result of deliberate efforts; continued intervention measures are required to prevent reintroduction.

Emphysema – a disorder affecting the alveoli (tiny air sacs) of the lungs. The transfer of oxygen and carbon dioxide in the lungs takes place in the walls of the alveoli. In emphysema, the alveoli become abnormally inflated, damaging their walls and making it harder to breathe. People who smoke or have chronic bronchitis have an increased risk of emphysema.

Equality – the term health inequalities is often used as a synonym for health inequities, but it is not, in that health inequalities are not always unfair. Equality can be assessed with respect to specified measurable outcomes, whereas judging whether a process is equitable or not is more open to interpretation. For example, young adults being healthier than the elderly population or men having prostate problems and women not, are health inequalities but not health inequities.

Equity – principle of being fair to all, with reference to a defined and recognized set of values. Equity in health implies that everyone should have a fair opportunity to attain their full health potential, and that no one should be disadvantaged from achieving this potential.

Eradication – permanent reduction to zero of the global incidence of infection as a result of deliberate efforts; intervention measures are no longer needed.

Famine – extensive food insecurity and food availability decline, wherein people have neither the entitlement nor physical and economic access to sufficient, safe, nutritious and culturally acceptable food to meet their dietary needs.

Fertility rate (total) – refers to the number of children that would be born per woman, given the persistence of current fertility rates and assuming no female mortality at childbearing ages.

Food fortification – the addition of a nutrient to a food. The food chosen as a carrier needs to be a good source to reach the target population.

Gametocytes – the sexual reproductive stage of malaria parasites. Gametocytes circulate in the blood stream, are picked up by the *Anopheles* mosquito, undergo sexual reproduction in the midgut of the mosquito, and attach to the mosquito's midgut, where they form an oocyst that eventually produces sporozoites.

Global Fund to fight AIDS, Tuberculosis and Malaria – a global public–private partnership created in 2002 and dedicated to attracting and disbursing additional financial resources to prevent and treat HIV/AIDS, tuberculosis and malaria.

Guinea worm – a threadlike worm (*Dracunculus medinensis*) of tropical Africa and Asia that is a subcutaneous parasite of humans and other mammals and that causes ulcerative lesions of the legs and feet.

Haemorrhage – bleeding or to lose blood. When this occurs from the female genital tract after 20 weeks of pregnancy it is called antepartum haemorrhage; excessive bleeding (usually more than 500 mls) after delivery is called post-partum haemorrhage.

Health systems – all organizations, people and actions whose primary intent is to promote, restore or maintain health.

Helminth – a large, multicellular organism ('worm') that is generally visible to the naked eye in its adult stages. Helminths can be free-living or parasitic.

Highly Active Antiretroviral Therapy (HAART) – a term used to describe anti-HIV combination therapy with three or more drugs.

Hookworm – parasitic nematode worm that lives in the small intestine of its host. Hookworms, if present in large numbers, can cause iron deficiency anaemia by sucking blood from the host's intestinal walls.

Hypertension – high blood pressure, defined as a repeatedly elevated blood pressure exceeding 140 over 90mm Hg – a systolic blood pressure above 140 with a diastolic blood pressure above 90.

Hypertension in pregnancy – might be chronic, already existing hypertension or pregnancy-induced (usually starts after 20 weeks of pregnancy). Both types of hypertension increase the risk of preeclampsia and eclampsia, and other causes of maternal mortality, including stroke and renal failure. Preeclampsia is hypertension in pregnancy plus protein loss in the urine, eclampsia is unexplained general seizures in patients with preeclampsia.

Incidence – indicates how often a disease or condition occurs. More precisely, it corresponds to the number of new cases of a disease or condition among a certain group of people for a certain period of time.

Indirect causes of maternal mortality – are those deaths resulting from previously existing disease or disease that developed during pregnancy and which was not directly the result of obstetric conditions, but which was aggravated by the physiological effects of the pregnancy.

Infant mortality rate – the number of deaths under one year of age occurring among the live births in a geographical area during a given year, expressed per 1000 live births.

Insulin – a hormone secreted by beta cells in the pancreas. Insulin plays a major role in the regulation of glucose metabolism, as well as being an important regulator of protein and lipid metabolism. Insulin is used as a drug to control insulin-dependant diabetes mellitus (type 1).

Intestinal obstruction – a mechanical or functional obstruction of the intestines, preventing the normal transit of the products of digestion.

Intestinal perforation – a hole in the intestinal wall, allowing intestinal contents to enter the abdominal cavity.

Intrauterine device ('IUD') – contraceptive device consisting of a piece (often T-shaped) of plastic or metal that is inserted through the vagina into the uterus.

Kaposi's Sarcoma – a type of cancer characterized by abnormal growth of blood vessels that develop into lesions of the skin and/or internal organs.

Kwashiorkor – form of childhood undernutrition characterized by oedema, irritability, anorexia, skin abnormalities and enlarged liver. The presence of oedema caused by poor nutrition defines kwashiorkor. The cause of kwashiorkor was thought to be due to insufficient protein consumption alone, however, micronutrient and antioxidant deficiencies in the presence of stressors like infection are associated with kwashiorkor and are now assumed to be of importance.

Leishmaniasis – a parasitic disease spread by the bite of a sand-fly infected with a protozoa (*Leishmania*). There are several forms of leishmaniasis, the most common being cutaneous and visceral leishmaniasis. The cutaneous form of the disease causes skin sores while the visceral form affects internal organs such as the spleen, liver and bone marrow and can be fatal.

Leprosy – a chronic infection caused by the bacterium *Mycobacterium leprae* which affects various parts of the body, including, in particular, the skin and nerves.

Life expectancy – the average number of years a group of people born in the same year can be expected to live assuming that mortality rates by age remain constant.

Loop electrosurgical excision procedure – entails the excision of the abnormal tissue with cauterization, utilizing a thin electrical wire in the form of a loop. Requires electricity, has higher costs, more technical expertise is needed compared to cryotherapy, and there is a higher risk of bleeding complications.

Low birthweight – infants born at weights under 2.5kg at birth are classified as having low birth weight.

Lymphatic filariasis – disease caused by thread-like parasitic worms, known as filariae, that lodge in the lymphatic system. Filariae are responsible for a variety of clinical manifestations, including lymphoedema of the limbs (elephantiasis), genital disease (including hydrocele) and acute, recurrent bacterial infections known as 'acute attacks'.

Macrophages – a type of white blood cells that begin their lives as monocytes. Monocytes are produced in the bone marrow and circulate throughout the blood stream. When an infection triggers a response, the monocytes can leave the blood stream and enter other tissues and organs in the body. After leaving the blood stream, monocytes develop into macrophages.

Marasmus – a form of undernutrition characterized by low weight for age and caused by chronic energy-deficiency. A child with marasmus looks emaciated with wasting of subcutaneous fat and muscles, and the bodyweight may reduce to less than 80 per cent of the normal weight for age.

Maternal mortality – is the death of a woman while pregnant or within 42 days of termination of pregnancy, irrespective of the duration and site of the pregnancy, from any cause related to or aggravated by the pregnancy or its management but not from accidental or incidental causes.

Maternal mortality ratio – shows the number of maternal deaths per 100,000 live births. This measure indicates the risk of maternal death among pregnant and recently pregnant women. It reflects a woman's basic health status, her access to health care and the quality of services that she receives.

Merozoites – daughter cells formed by asexual development in the life cycle of malaria parasites. Liver-stage and blood-stage malaria parasites develop into schizonts which contain many merozoites. When the schizonts are mature, they (and their host cells) rupture, the merozoites are released and infect red blood cells.

Micro-health insurance – a form of health insurance, which offers limited protection at a low contribution (hence the term 'micro'). It is aimed at the poor and designed to help them cover themselves collectively against catastrophic health expenditure. Often these schemes are linked to community and civil society groups.

Millennium Development Goals – the goals endorsed by governments at the United Nations in September 2000. These aim to improve human well-being by reducing poverty, hunger, child and maternal mortality, ensuring education for all, controlling and managing diseases, tackling gender-disparity, ensuring sustainable development and pursuing global partnerships.

Multidrug resistant tuberculosis (MDR-TB) – active tuberculosis caused by *Mycobacterium tuberculosis* organisms that are resistant to more than one anti-tuberculosis drug; in practice this often refers to organisms that are resistant to both isoniazid and rifampicin. Essentially, MDR-TB is a resistance to nearly all medicines used to treat tuberculosis.

Mycobacterium tuberculosis – the bacterium that causes tuberculosis. *M. tuberculosis* has unusually waxy walls, is slow-growing and amongst the most recalcitrant bacteria to treatment.

Neonatal deaths – deaths among live births during the first 28 days of life.

Nuclear magnetic resonance scan – the use of magnetic fields and radio waves (instead of X-rays used in CAT scans) to visualize body structures and how they function.

Obesity – excess body fat. Because body fat is usually not measured, a ratio of body weight to height, expressed as the body mass index (BMI; weight in kilograms/height in meters^2), is often used instead. An adult who has a BMI of 30 or higher is considered obese.

Onchocerciasis – also known as river blindness, is the world's second most common infectious cause of blindness. It is caused by *Onchocerca volvulus*, a worm that can live up to 15 years in the human body. It is transmitted to the human body through the bite of a blackfly (*Simulium*).

The worms spread out through the body, and when they die, they cause intense itching and a strong immune response that can destroy nearby tissue, such as the eye.

Oocysts – oocysts are *Plasmodium* cysts located in the outer wall of the mosquito midgut or stomach, where sporozoite development takes place. When mature, the oocysts rupture and release sporozoites. Sporozoites, which are delicate spindle-shaped stages, migrate via the haemocoel to the mosquito's salivary gland, and are injected into the host when the mosquito feeds.

Oral contraceptive pills – birth control pills that contain hormones (usually synthetic oestrogen and progestin) that prevent the ovaries from releasing an egg. Even if an egg is released, birth control pills make it difficult for sperm to fertilize the egg.

Palliative care – the total care of patients with progressive, incurable illness. In palliative care, the focus of care is on the quality of life. Control of pain and other physical symptoms, and addressing psychological, social and spiritual problems is considered most important.

Parasite – organism that derives benefit from another organism. The other organism is usually termed the 'host' and the action of the parasite is usually detrimental to the host. There are many protozoan and helminth parasites of medical importance.

Partograph – is a written record charting the progress of labour and delivery and showing the key observations to monitor the mother, the foetus and progression of labour.

Pellagra – disease caused by deficiency of niacin (vitamin B3). Symptoms include diarrhoea, skin inflammation (dermatitis) and dementia. If left untreated death is the usual outcome.

PEPFAR – launched in 2003, the US President's Emergency Plan For AIDS Relief aims to combat HIV/AIDS, and claims to be the largest commitment by any nation to combat a single disease in history.

Plasmodium – the genus of the protozoan parasite that causes malaria. The genus includes four species that infect humans: *Plasmodium falciparum*, *Plasmodium vivax*, *Plasmodium ovale*, and *Plasmodium malariae*. Quite recently, thousands of people in South East Asia have been found naturally infected with a monkey malaria *Plasmodium knowlesi* so this should now be considered as the fifth human malaria species.

Pneumocystis carinii – fungus that causes pneumonia, and occurs in immunosupressed individuals and in premature, malnourished infants. New term is *pneumocystis jiroveci*.

Prevalence – the proportion of individuals who at a particular time (be it a point in time or time period) have a disease or condition.

Protectionism – protection of a domestic industry from cheaper competitive imports by such means as import duties, import quotas, export subsidies, health and environmental regulations.

Protozoa – single-celled, microscopic organisms that can perform all necessary functions of metabolism and reproduction. Some protozoa are free-living, while others parasitize other organisms for their nutrients and life cycle

Pyrethroids – a class of insecticides derived from natural pyrethrins.

Quinine – a drug used against malaria, obtained from the bark of the cinchona tree.

Randomized controlled trial – a study in which subjects are assigned by chance to receive one of several clinical interventions. The people in the study are as much alike as possible at the onset of the trial and are cared for in the same way throughout the trial. Any differences can then be attributed to the differences in interventions alone, and not to bias or chance.

Residual insecticide spraying – treatment of houses where people spend their night-time hours, by spraying insecticides that have a residual effect (i.e. that continue to affect mosquitoes for several months). Residual insecticide spraying aims to kill mosquitoes when they come to rest on the walls, usually after a blood meal.

Rhythm method – also called natural family planning, rhythm is a method of birth control that focuses on learning to recognize the days a woman is fertile, and abstaining from sex before and during those days.

Rickets – disease caused by a deficiency of vitamin D with disturbance of normal ossification in infants and children. The disease is marked by bending and distortion of the bones under muscular action, by the formation of nodular enlargements at the ends and sides of the bones, by delayed closure of the fontanels, and pain in the muscles.

RNA – ribonucleic acid. One of the two types of nucleic acid found in all cells, the other one being DNA. RNA transmits genetic information from DNA to proteins produced by the cell.

Scabies – infestation of the skin by the human itch mite, *Sarcoptes scabiei*. The initial symptoms of scabies are red, raised bumps that are intensely itchy. A magnifying glass will reveal short, wavy lines of red skin, which are burrows made by the mites.

Schistosomiasis – also known as bilharzia or snail fever, is a parasitic disease carried by fresh water snails with one of the five species of the parasite *Schistosoma*. Urinary schistosomiasis causes scarring and tearing of the bladder and kidneys, and can lead to bladder cancer. Intestinal schistosomiasis can result in enlargement of the liver, lungs and spleen, and can cause abdominal bleeding and damage to the intestines.

Schizonts – developmental forms of the malaria parasites that contain many merozoites. Schizonts are seen in the liver-stage and blood-stage parasites.

Scurvy – disease caused by a deficiency of ascorbic acid (vitamin C). Symptoms include weakness, softening and bleeding of the gums, peri-ostal bleeding and pain in joints and muscles, and abnormal bone and tooth growth.

Sensitivity – refers to the extent to which a test is capable of correctly diagnosing the presence of the disease concerned. It is expressed as the proportion of people with the disease who have a positive test result.

Social health insurance – a scheme where potential participants are obliged or encouraged to be insured. For example, a government may oblige all employees to participate in a social security programme; employers may make it a condition of employment that employees participate in an insurance programme specified by the employer; an employer may encourage employees to join a programme by making contributions on behalf of the employee; or a trade union may arrange advantageous insurance cover available only to the members of the trade union.

Social marketing – the use of commercial marketing techniques to achieve a social objective. In global health, social marketing programmes have focused on increasing the availability and use of health products, such as insecticide treated bed nets or contraceptives.

Specificity – refers to the extent to which the test is capable of correctly diagnosing the absence of the disease concerned. It is expressed as the proportion of people without the disease who have a negative test result.

Sporozoites – the infective stage of the malaria parasite that is passed to the human host from the salivary glands of the mosquito. Sporozoites infect liver cells, disappearing from the bloodstream within 30 minutes. The mechanism for this amazingly rapid disappearance from the bloodstream to the liver is still unknown.

Staging in oncology – the process of categorizing a tumor in terms of its size, its degree of invasion into surrounding tissue and its spread to nearby lymph nodes.

Structural adjustment programmes – economic policies for low- and middle-income countries that have been promoted by the World Bank and the International Monetary Fund since the early 1980s by the provision of loans conditional on the adoption of such policies. The programmes were designed to bring about open markets, liberalized trade and to lower government budget and current account deficits.

Stunting – low height for age, reflecting a sustained past episode or episodes of undernutrition and growth faltering.

Trachoma – infectious disease of the eye caused by the bacterium *Chlamydia trachomatis*. Repeated exposure to the disease over time eventually causes the inside of the eyelid to turn inward – a condition called trichiasis – and the eyelashes to scrape and scar the cornea, leading to blindness.

Trichiasis – one or more eyelashes touching the eye due to trachoma-related scarring of the lids.

Trichurias – the human whipworm, *Trichuris trichuria*, is an intestinal parasite. Symptoms of trichurias infection can include diarrhoea, dysentery and anaemia.

Typhoid – infectious fever usually spread by food, milk or water supplies that have been affected by the bacterium *Salmonella typhi*, either directly by sewage, indirectly by flies or as a result of poor personal hygiene.

Under-five-mortality rate – the probability of dying between birth and 5 years of age, expressed as a rate per 1000 live births. It is otherwise known as the child mortality rate.

Undernutrition – the result of inadequate food intake and repeated infectious diseases. Includes being underweight for one's age, too short for one's age (stunting), too thin for one's age (wasting) and deficient in vitamins and minerals (micronutrient deficiency).

Underweight – low weight for age in children, and Body Mass Index < 18.5 in adults, reflecting a current condition from inadequate food intake, past episodes of undernutrition or poor health condition.

User fees – charges for health care at the point of use; user fees were introduced in poor countries for public services in health and education on the direction of the World Bank and other donors in the 1980s–1990s to tackle severe under-funding.

Varicose veins – a dilated (widened) tortuous (twisting) vein, usually involving a superficial vein in the leg, often associated with incompetency of the valves in the vein. These visible and bulging veins are often associated with symptoms such as tired, heavy or aching legs.

Verbal autopsy – a process used to collect information using a specially-designed series of questions from relatives or caregivers of a deceased person. The process involves interviewing relatives or caregivers regarding their observations and descriptions of the symptoms, signs and circumstances leading to the death. The information that is collected is used by medical personnel to assign a probable cause of death.

Vesicovaginal fistula – is an abnormal opening between the bladder and the vagina that results in continuous and unremitting urinary incontinence.

Wasting – characterized by the 'shrivelled' child, often caused by either acute or chronic energy deficiency and expressed in low weight for height.

Yellow fever – an acute systematic illness caused by a virus called *Flavivirus*. In severe cases, the viral infection causes a high fever, bleeding into the skin, and necrosis (death) of cells in the kidney and liver. The damage done in the liver from the virus results in severe jaundice which yellows the skin.

Index